SUBSTANCE ABUSE

Recent Titles in
A World View of Social Issues Series

SUBSTANCE ABUSE

A GLOBAL VIEW

Edited by Andrew Cherry,
Mary E. Dillon, and
Douglas Rugh

A World View of Social Issues

Greenwood Press
Westport, Connecticut • London

Library of Congress Cataloging-in-Publication Data

Substance abuse : a global view / edited by Andrew Cherry . . . [et al.].
    p. cm.—(A world view of social issues, ISSN 1526–9442)
    Includes bibliographical references and index.
    ISBN 0–313–31218–4 (alk. paper)
    1. Drug abuse. 2. Substance abuse. I. Cherry, Andrew L. II. Series.
HV5801.S834 2002
    362.29—dc21   2001033684

British Library Cataloguing in Publication Data is available.

Library of Congress Catalog Card Number: 2001033684
ISBN: 0–313–31218–4
ISSN: 1526–9442

First published in 2002

Greenwood Press, 88 Post Road West, Westport, CT 06881
An imprint of Greenwood Publishing Group, Inc.
www.greenwood.com

Printed in the United States of America

The paper used in this book complies with the
Permanent Paper Standard issued by the National
Information Standards Organization (Z39.48–1984).

10 9 8 7 6 5 4 3 2 1

CONTENTS

SERIES FOREWORD

Why are child abuse in the family and homelessness social conditions to be endured or at least tolerated in some countries while in other countries they are viewed as social problems that must be reduced or eliminated? What social institutions and other factors affect these behaviors? What historical, political, and social forces influence a society's response to a social condition? In many cases, individuals around the world have the same or similar hopes and problems. However, in most cases we deal with the same social conditions in very dissimilar ways.

The volumes in the Greenwood series A World View of Social Issues examine different social issues and problems that are being faced by individuals and societies around the world. These volumes examine problems of poverty and homelessness, drugs and alcohol addiction, HIV/AIDS, teen pregnancy, crime, women's rights, and a myriad of other issues that affect all of us in one way or another.

Each volume is devoted to one social issue or problem. All volumes follow the same general format. Each volume has up to fifteen chapters that describe how people in different countries perceive and try to cope with a given problem or social issue. The countries chosen represent as many world regions as possible, making it possible to explore how each issue has been recognized and what actions have been taken to alleviate it in a variety of settings.

Each chapter begins with a profile of the country being highlighted and an overview of the impact of the social issue or problem there. Basic policies, legislation, and demographic information related to the social issue are covered. A brief history of the problem helps the reader better understand the political and social responses. Political initiatives and policies are also discussed, as well as social views, customs, and practices related to the problem or social issue. Discussions about how the countries plan to deal with these social problems are also included.

These volumes present a comprehensive and engaging approach for the study of international social conditions and problems. The goal is to provide a convenient framework for readers to examine specific social problems, how they are viewed, and what actions are being taken by different countries around the world.

For example, how is a problem like crime and crime control handled in third world countries? How is substance abuse controlled in industrialized countries? How are poverty and homelessness handled in the poorest countries? How does culture influence the definition, and response to, domestic violence in different countries? What part does economics play in shaping both the issue of and the response to women's rights? How does a national philosophy impact the definition of and response to child abuse? These questions and more will be answered by the volumes in this series.

As we learn more about our counterparts in other countries, they become real to us, and our worldview cannot help but change. We will think of others as we think of those we know. They will be people who get up in the morning and go to work. We will see people who are struggling with relationships, attending religious services, being born, and growing old, and dying.

This series will cover issues that will add to your knowledge about contemporary social society. These volumes will help you to better understand social conditions and social issues in a broader sense, giving you a view of what various problems mean to different people and how these perspectives impact a society's response. You will be able to see how specific social problems are managed by governments and individuals confronting the consequences of these social dilemmas. By studying one problem from various angles, you will be better able to grasp the totality of the situation, while at the same time speculating as to how solutions used in one country could be incorporated in another. Finally, this series will allow you to compare and contrast how these social issues impact individuals in different countries and how the effect is dissimilar or similar to your own experiences.

As series adviser, it is my hope that these volumes, which are unique in the history of publishing, will increase your understanding and appreciation of your counterparts around the world.

Andrew Cherry
Series Adviser

INTRODUCTION

The global drug problem has three major themes, which are clearly discernible in most countries around the world: concern about young people and drugs; concern about addiction; and concern about the effects of the illegal production, trafficking, and selling of drugs. Two major policy and programming approaches are used to deal with these three primary concerns about drug use: the criminal justice model, which is used to stop or control drug use; and the public health model, based on harm reduction, which is used to reduce the health problems among drug users that are caused by the drugs they use. The best example of the prohibition model is China, and the best example of the harm reduction model is the Netherlands, although all countries use some combination of these drug-control strategies.

When the drug-abuse problem is examined on a global scale, it becomes clear how the production, trafficking, and retailing of illegal drugs affect addiction as well as public and social policy. The production of drugs falls into three categories: those processes requiring only plant products (cannabis and raw opium); those processes involving a semi-synthetic process in which natural materials are partly changed by synthetic substances to produce the final product (coca bush leaves processed to make cocaine); and those using only manmade chemicals to produce consumable drugs (narcotic or psychotropic drugs, such as LSD, made entirely in the laboratory or factory).

DEFINITIONS

Drug addiction, or drug abuse, is a chronic or habitual use of any chemical substance to alter states of the mind for any purpose other than a medically warranted one. Traditional definitions of addiction, with their criteria of physical dependence and withdrawal (and often an underlying tenor of depravity and sin), have been modified with increased understanding; with the introduction of new drugs, such as cocaine, which are psychologically or neuropsychologically addicting; and with the realization that its stereotypical application to opiate-drug users was invalid because many opiate users remain occasional users with no physical dependence. Today addiction is more often defined by the continuing, compulsive nature of the drug use despite physical and psychological harm to the user and society, and it includes both licit and illicit drugs. The term "substance abuse" is now frequently used because of the broad range of substances (including alcohol and inhalants) which fit the addictive profile. Psychological dependence is the subjective feeling that the user needs the drug to maintain a feeling of well-being; physical dependence is characterized by tolerance (the need for increasingly larger doses to feed the addiction) and withdrawal symptoms experienced when the user practices abstinence.

Definitions of drug abuse and addiction are subjective and are infused with the political and moral values of the society and culture. For example, the stimulant caffeine is a drug used by millions of people in coffee and tea. Because of the relatively mild stimulatory effects of caffeine and because caffeine typically does not trigger antisocial behavior in users, the drinking of coffee and tea, despite the fact that caffeine is physically addictive, is not generally considered drug abuse. In certain social contexts, even narcotics addiction can be regarded as only drug abuse. In India, for example, opium has been used for centuries without becoming unduly corrosive to the social fabric.

DRUG RESEARCH AND INFORMATION

The illegality of the drug trade, which was established by a public policy of prohibition, has resulted in an environment characterized by secrecy and danger. The legality issue is one of the most important factors determining the forms in which drugs are produced, transported, sold, and consumed. It is also an extremely significant factor in drug pricing. Danger and secrecy also present significant methodological difficulties for would-be students in drug trafficking; this may explain why so much drug research has been focused on policy.

Money is another crucial element that explains why so much research has focused on policy. Indeed, on the average, the federal government has spent well over $10 billion a year on drug control for at least the last ten years. Currently, fifty-two federal agencies have a stake in drug control, and each must justify its budget. The sharing of the national drug-control "cake"— that is, the annual allocation of funds by Congress—generates a bureaucratic and public debate in which arguments are used to support requests for funds (Baum, 1996; Bureau of Justice Statistics, 2000).

EFFECTS ON THE INDIVIDUAL

People who use drugs [→ Cocaine] experience a wide array of physical effects other than those expected. (The excitement of a cocaine high, for instance, is followed by a "crash": a period of anxiety, fatigue, depression, and an acute desire for more cocaine to alleviate the feelings of the crash.) Alcohol, which interferes with motor control, is a factor in many automobile accidents. Users of marijuana and hallucinogenic drugs may experience unwanted recurrences of the drug's effects weeks or months after use. Sudden abstinence from certain drugs results in withdrawal symptoms. Heroin withdrawal can cause vomiting, muscle cramps, convulsions, and delirium. Increased sexual activity among drug users, both in prostitution and from the disinhibiting effect of some drugs, puts users at a higher risk of contracting AIDS and other sexually transmitted diseases.

Because the purity and dosage of illegal drugs are uncontrolled, drug overdose is a constant risk. More than 10,000 deaths annually in the United States are directly attributable to drug use. The most frequently involved substances are cocaine, heroin, and morphine, often in combination with alcohol or other drugs (Bureau of Justice Statistics, 2000). Many drug users engage in criminal activity, such as burglary and prostitution, to raise the money to buy drugs; some drugs, especially alcohol, PCP, and cocaine, are associated with violent behavior.

EFFECTS ON THE FAMILY

A problem more common in the United States and other developed countries is the drug user's preoccupation with the substance, as well as its effects on mood and performance, which can lead to marital problems and poor work performance or job dismissal. Drug use can disrupt family life and create destructive patterns of codependency. The spouse, or the whole family, out of love or fear of the consequences, may inadvertently enable the user to continue using drugs by covering up, by supplying money, or by denying a problem exists. Pregnant drug users, because of the drugs themselves or poor self-care in general, bear a much higher rate of low birth-weight babies than the average. Many drugs, including crack and heroin, cross the placental barrier, resulting in addicted babies who go through withdrawal soon after birth. Fetal alcohol syndrome can affect children of mothers who consume alcohol during pregnancy. Pregnant women who acquire the AIDS virus through intravenous drug use pass the virus on to their infants.

EFFECTS ON SOCIETY

Drug abuse affects society in many ways. In the United States, it is costly in terms of its effect in the workplace, including lost work time and inefficiency. Drug users are more likely than nonusers to have occupational accidents, endangering themselves and those around them. Almost 40 percent of the highway deaths in the United States involve alcohol. Drug-related crime can disrupt neighborhoods with violence among the drug dealers themselves, threats to residents, and the crimes committed by the addicts. In some neighborhoods, younger children are recruited as lookouts and helpers because of the lighter sentences given to juvenile offenders. Hence, guns have become commonplace among children and adolescents in many inner-city communities in the United States. The great majority of homeless people have either a drug or alcohol problem or a mental illness; many have both (Voas and Tippetts, 1999).

TREATMENT

For every person undergoing drug treatment in the United States, there are an estimated three or four people who need treatment. Many who attempt to get treatment, especially from public facilities, are discouraged by waits of over a month to get into treatment. Evaluating the effectiveness of a treatment program is difficult because of the chronic nature of drug abuse and alcoholism and the fact that the disease is usually complicated by personal, social, and health factors.

LEGALIZATION AND DECRIMINALIZATION

The concept of controlling drugs is a relatively recent phenomenon, and one that has been met with limited success despite the billions of dollars spent. Some people argue that if drugs were legalized (as occurred with the repeal of Prohibition in the 1930s), drug trafficking and its concomitant violence would disappear. Some contend that with government regulation, dosages for addicts would be standardized and dangerous contaminants would be eliminated, making the drugs safer. It has also been suggested that the resulting lower prices for drugs would preclude the need for criminal activity to raise money for their purchase; the low prices would drive traffickers out of business; and the billions of dollars saved from supply-reduction programs could be used for drug education and treatment. Nevertheless, a substantial majority of Americans in the year 2000 continued to view drugs and drug use as intrinsically bad. Those opposed to legalization believe that removal of deterrents would encourage drug use, that people would still steal to buy drugs, and that many drugs are so inexpensive to produce that there would still be a black market.

Decriminalization is the elimination or reduction of criminal penalties for using or dealing in small amounts of certain drugs. Attitudes toward decriminalization change with the times and with actual and perceived dangers involved. Many localities decriminalized marijuana in the 1970s—and many reinstituted stricter laws in the 1980s (Abadinsky, 1997).

HISTORY

Humans have used drugs of various sorts for thousands of years. Beer was consumed as long ago as the time of the early Egyptians; narcotics have been used since 4000 B.C.; and the earliest medicinal use of marijuana has been dated to 2737 B.C. in China. However, not until the nineteenth century A.D. were the active substances in these drugs extracted or understood. There followed a time when some of these newly discovered substances—morphine, laudanum, and cocaine—were completely unregulated and prescribed freely by physicians, pharmacists, and other healers for a wide variety of ailments. They were available in patent medicines and sold by traveling tinkers, in drugstores, or through the mail. During the American Civil War, morphine was used freely, and wounded veterans returned home with their kits of morphine and hypodermic needles. Opium dens flourished. By the early 1900s, there were an estimated 250,000 addicts in the United States (Brecher, 1972).

The problems of addiction were recognized only gradually. Legal measures against drug abuse in the United States were first established in 1875, when opium dens were outlawed in San Francisco. The first national drug law, the Pure Food and Drug Act of 1906, required accurate labeling of patent medicines containing opium and certain other drugs. In 1914, the Harrison Narcotic Act forbade the sale of substantial doses of opiates or cocaine except by licensed doctors and pharmacies. Later, heroin was totally banned. Subsequent U.S. Supreme Court decisions made it illegal for doctors to prescribe any narcotic to addicts; doctors who prescribed maintenance doses as part of an addiction treatment plan were jailed, and soon all attempts at treatment were abandoned. The use of narcotics and cocaine had diminished by the 1920s. The spirit of temperance led to the prohibition of alcohol by the Eighteenth Amendment to the U.S. Constitution in 1919, but Prohibition was repealed in 1933 (Brecher, 1972).

In the 1930s, most states required antidrug education in the schools, but fears that knowledge would lead to experimentation caused it to be abandoned in most places. Soon after the repeal of Prohibition, the U.S. Federal Bureau of Narcotics (now the Drug Enforcement Administration) began a campaign to portray marijuana as a powerful, addicting substance that would lead users into narcotics addiction. In the 1950s, use of marijuana increased again, along with that of amphetamines and tranquilizers. The social upheaval of the 1960s brought with it a dramatic increase in drug use and some increased social acceptance; by the early 1970s, some states and localities had decriminalized marijuana and lowered drinking ages. The 1980s brought a decline in the use of most drugs, but cocaine and crack use soared. The military became involved in border patrols for the first time, and troops invaded Panama and brought its de facto leader, Manuel Noriega, to trial for drug trafficking (Massing, 1998).

Throughout the years, the public's perception of the dangers of specific substances has changed. The surgeon general's warning label on tobacco packaging gradually made people aware of the addictive nature of nicotine. By 1995 the Food and Drug Administration was considering regulating tobacco. The recognition of fetal alcohol syndrome brought warning labels to alcohol products. The addictive nature of prescription drugs such as diazepam (Valium) became known, and caffeine came under scrutiny as well (Jonnes, 1999).

In the United States, as in other countries, drug laws have been changed to keep up with the varying perceptions and real dangers of substance abuse. By 1970 countless state laws specified a variety of punitive measures, including life imprisonment and even the death penalty. To streamline these laws, the Comprehensive Drug Abuse Prevention and Control Act of 1970 repealed, replaced, or updated all previous federal laws concerned with narcotics and all other dangerous drugs. Possession was made illegal, but the severest penalties were reserved for illicit distribution and manufacture of drugs (Jonnes, 1999). But, like the Hydra, as a threatening head of the drug problem was cut off, two equally threatening heads or drug problems emerged from the same neck.

Chapter 9 on Mexico is included here to illustrate the effect on a small, poor, but proud and defiant country caught between a rich giant nation with a tremendous drug appetite and drug producers. Colombia (Chapter 4) is a good illustration of how a group of quasi-businessmen who became involved in trafficking marijuana and cocaine became the biggest and richest cartel in the world with an estimated wealth of $100 billion. The illegal drug trade is estimated to bring in $400 billion a year worldwide.

DRUGS AND THE WORLD'S YOUTH

One of the primary concerns of the global drug problem is the impact on the young people who are at a stage in life where they are trying to assert their independence. They are more willing to take risks. All common adult experiences are new to young people growing into adulthood. Drugs, coffee, cigarettes, alcohol, marijuana, heroin, cocaine, and drugs like Ecstasy are a part of the adolescent world, whether they experiment with them or use them. Each adolescent must develop a personal strategy for avoiding addiction.

What is the best approach for accomplishing this goal? The harm-reduction model has the best record to date. While the harm-reduction model, as it is used in the Netherlands, does not view abstinence as a necessary goal, it supports the idea. Outcomes that can be expected from a harm-reduction model, compared to nations that use a prohibition model, would include drug initiation occurring later in age, fewer young people experimenting with hard drugs, and the initiation to hard drugs occurring later in age.

Figure I.1
Lifetime Prevalence of the Use of Hard Drugs among Youth between
Fourteen and Twenty Years of Age

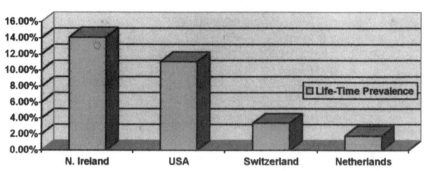

Source: Killias and Ribeaud, 1999.

International data collected from twelve countries about juvenile drug use
and crime provide information that can be used to draw conclusions about
the prohibition and the harm-reduction models (International Juv-
CrimeDgs). Based on the data available on the countries included in the
chapters in this book, a lifetime prevalence of hard drugs (heroin, cocaine,
crack, amphetamines, Ecstasy, LSD, and so on) is very important in determining future addiction. Figure I.1 shows the difference in the lifetime use
of hard drugs for people between the ages of fourteen and twenty.

Another very important issue related to youth who use drugs is the age
of initiation. The later the age of initiation, the less chance a person has of
becoming addicted when experimentation with drugs occurs. In Figure I.2,
the country with the lowest average initiation rate is the United States,
which has the lowest initiation age on all three drugs (alcohol, soft drugs,
and hard drugs). The United States is also the country with the most active
prohibition model of drug control. In the countries where drugs have been
more or less decriminalized the age of initiation is much older. Starting to
experiment with drugs a year or two later than the average (in terms of drug
experimentation) can save many young people the misery of addiction and
save society both human resources and the money that would be spent to
deal with an addict over his or her lifetime. Furthermore, when there is little
difference between the age of the first use of a soft drug and the age of the
first use of a hard drug, typically, the adolescent drug user is buying both
the soft drug and the hard drug from the same source. This is a very effective
way to addict as many youths as possible to hard drugs.

GLOBAL DRUG ABUSE

Three reports, published by the United Nations Drugs Control and Crime
Prevention program provide an insight into the global spread of drug abuse.

Figure I.2
Average Age at First Use of Alcohol and Drugs among Youth between
Fourteen and Twenty Years of Age

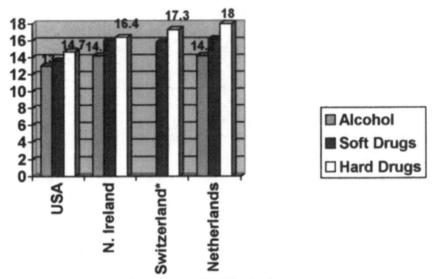

*No data for age of alcohol onset reported by Switzerland.
Source: Killias and Ribeaud, 1999.

In the language of statistics, they provide an overview of the scale and depth of drug use internationally.

These reports reveal that the illegal drug business accounts for $400 billion of world trade, and is second only to the worldwide arms market (ODCCP, 2000). It is larger than the global iron and steel industries. The 2000 *World Drug Report* noted that there were at least 180 million drug abusers globally, including 9 million heroin addicts, 29 million amphetamine users, and 14 million cocaine users (ODCCP, 2000).

In the report called *Global Illicit Drug Trends* (1999), many of the world's opiate and cocaine addicts can be found close to the illicit drug producing areas where half of all opium and cocaine is consumed. In some producing areas, in Iran, between 4 and 6 percent of the population are opium addicts. The country has an estimated 1.2 million opiate addicts, including 150,000 heroin users. In the producing areas of Laos and Thailand, the addiction rate is as high as 10 percent. Fully 80 percent of the heroin consumed in Europe comes via the Balkans. Of the opium that comes from Southeast Asia, as much as 50 percent is sent to China. In the United States and Canada, in 1991 there were 360,000 heroin addicts; in 2000 there were 600,000 heroin addicts. In the United Kingdom, Ireland,

Denmark, and Italy, 2 percent of 16- and 17-year-olds have used heroin (ODCCP, 1999b).

Worldwide, 11 percent of AIDS cases are estimated to be a result of drug users injecting themselves with dirty needles, particularly heroin addicts. Countries reporting a rise in injection between 1996 and 1998 noted a 37 percent increase in HIV infection (ODCCP, 1999b).

In recent years, use and production of cocaine have increased. World production is centered on Latin America: Colombia (56%), Peru (28%), and Bolivia (16%). Together, these countries produce nearly 180,000 tons of coca leaf. In 1998 eradication programs destroyed 98,630 hectares of coca leaf crops, up from 3,446 hectares in 1986. The street price of cocaine averages $110 a gram. Most Latin American cocaine is sent to the United States, although some reaches Europe. Over 6 percent of America's young people have used cocaine, or its "crack" variant; in the Bahamas the number is 6.4 percent, and 4.5 percent in Kenya. Many people in drug-growing areas use raw coca leaf itself, or other unrefined cocaine products (ODCCP, 1999b).

By far the most ubiquitous drug is cannabis. It is estimated that over 140 million people regularly use cannabis worldwide. Among young adults, usage is far higher—37 percent in the United Kingdom for example. Thirty-eight countries reported an increase in cannabis use in the 1990s (ODCCP, 2000).

SUPPLY AND USAGE IN AFRICA

"The African Drug Nexus" (1999) report shows that the increased prevalence of drug abuse is a clear indicator of the drastic social and psychological damage produced by deepening poverty, social upheaval, and civil war. The report was compiled from questionnaires sent to various drug agencies in Cameroon, Côte d'Ivoire, Ghana, Ethiopia, Kenya, Mozambique, Nigeria, Senegal, South Africa, and Zimbabwe. Comments from both the UNDCP and the School of Oriental and African Studies in the University of London were also included. The countries surveyed are among the poorest in the world. Ethiopia has a per capita GDP of $450, Mozambique $810, Nigeria $1220, Cameroon $2,110, South Africa $5,030 (ODCCP, 1999a).

The report establishes that poor people use the most drugs. Unemployed people make up a large proportion of cannabis users. Of 553 drug users arrested in Ethiopia between 1993 and 1997, 50 percent were unemployed (ODCCP, 1999a).

Africa has huge youth populations—in Côte d'Ivoire more than half the entire population is under eighteen—and there is a growth in the numbers of "street children." There are 12,000 street children in the Ethiopian capital, Addis Ababa, alone. Among street children, qaat (a leaf that is chewed for stimulant effect), cannabis, and solvent abuse are the norm (ODCCP, 1999a).

A bewildering array of other substances are also used—from traditional cannabis infusions and hallucinogenics administered by faith healers, to Mandrax (the trade name for methaqualone, a barbiturate known in the U.S. as quaaludes) and beer mixes, petrol and solvents for inhalation, prescription medicine abuse, and crack cocaine.

In Kenya, chewing qaat is culturally acceptable. Because it causes insomnia, users need other drugs like cannabis to fall asleep. One survey of young Kenyans suggested that 63 percent regularly used drugs. Qaat is also widely used in Ethiopia. Fully 82 percent of Addis Ababa street children use some sort of drugs in a country with just one drug rehabilitation unit. Over 43 percent of mental patients are qaat addicts (ODCCP, 1999a).

The many urban slum areas with their poverty, tension, crime, overcrowding and lack of privacy create a fertile environment for the illegal drug industry. Many turn to drug dealing and other areas of "informal trade." The black market economy is the fastest growing area of the Ghanaian economy. Over 60 percent of the Senegalese GDP is "informal," employing 700,000 people, 45 percent of whom live in the capital city of Dakar (ODCCP, 1999a).

The fall in the world price of basic commodities has encouraged this shift to drug production. Côte d'Ivoire is the world's leading cocoa bean producer. In the 1990s, cocoa accounted for 50 percent of the GDP, and 4.8 million people, 40 percent of the population, depended on it for their livelihoods. Between 1988 and 1992, the price of cocoa fell by 50 percent: the country's credit system collapsed, and the planters' revenues fell by 60 percent. Two-thirds of the farmers interviewed said they started growing cannabis after the cocoa price collapse. One-tenth of an acre devoted to cannabis can yield the same profit as between thirty and forty acres devoted to cocoa (ODCCP, 2000).

The following chapters illustrate that each country has its own story of substance abuse, just as all countries have commonalities and similar drug problem experiences. The countries chosen for inclusion in this volume are all countries where the problem has been recognized and where different methods have been implemented in order to control it. At the beginning of the twenty-first century, most pragmatic researchers have given up on the prohibition model as a viable vehicle for ending drug abuse. At best, the prohibition model can be used to reduce trafficking. However, when a harm-reduction model, which supplies the abused drug to the addict, is used, the price of the drug is driven down so low that, like in any other supply-and-demand market, the trafficker goes out of business. Would that not be a novel conclusion?

REFERENCES

Abadinsky, H. (1997). *Drug abuse: An introduction* (3rd edition). Chicago: Nelson Hall.

Baum, D. (1996). *Smoke and mirrors: The war on drugs and the politics of failure.* Boston, MA: Little Brown and Company.

Brecher, E.M. (1972). *Licit and illicit drugs.* Boston: Little Brown and Company.

Bureau of Justice Statistics. (2000). *Drug law: Drug control budget U.S. 1981–2000.* Washington, D.C. U.S. Department of Justice.

Jonnes, J. (1999). *Hepcats, narcs, and pipe dreams: A history of America's romance with illegal drugs.* Washington, D.C.: Publications of the Drugs and Crime Data Center and Clearinghouse, the Bureau of Justice Statistics Clearinghouse, and the National Clearinghouse for Alcohol and Drug Information.

Killias, M. and Ribeaud, D. (1999). Drug use and crime among juveniles. An international perspective. *Studies on Crime and Crime Prevention, 8* (2), pp. 189–209.

Massing, M. (1998). *The fix.* New York: Simon and Schuster.

ODCCP [United Nations Office for Drug Control and Crime Prevention]. (1999a). *Drug nexus in Africa.* Vienna, Austria: United Nations.

ODCCP (1999b). *Global illicit drugs trends.* Vienna, Austria: United Nations.

ODCCP (2000). *World drug report.* Vienna, Austria: United Nations.

Voas, R.B., Tippetts, A.S. (1999, April). *The relationship of alcohol safety laws to drunk drivers in fatal crashes.* Washington, D.C.: National Highway Traffic and Safety Administration.

1

BURMA (UNION OF MYANMAR)

Andrew Cherry

INTRODUCTION

Burma, as this country has been known for hundreds of years, is like a natural jewel—rough on the exterior but with great beauty under the unpolished surface. It is a country of people who belong to more than one hundred different ethnic groups. Many of these ethnic groups live in virtual isolation from the Burmans, who constitute the largest ethnic group and the majority in Burma (Open Society Institute, 2000). The minority ethnic groups in Burma, who struggle for their very lives, use opium and heroin to finance the fight for their existence. For these rebels without a voice or a platform to plead their case, terrorism, drugs, arms, and civil corruption rule the day.

In the world community, Burma, or the Union of Myanmar (the name preferred by the current military government), has a very negative image. Burma represents the worst of the drug-producing countries in the world. The majority of the countries of the world have turned their backs on Burma. Other countries condemn Burma's involvement in opium poppy cultivation and heroin production. Burma has been boycotted by countries that have tried to stop the heroin from pouring out of Burma into their own countries. In the United States there are an estimated 600,000 heroin addicts, and 80 percent of the heroin used by these U.S. addicts comes from Burma (Agence France Presse, 1996). By blaming Burma for our problems, the rest of us can deny any complicity in the creation of Burma's drug-producing economy. Other countries feel justified in being repulsed by

Burma; others take advantage of the situation but have no remorse because Burma is the "bad" country.

The world community uses this rationale to blame Burma for the world heroin problem. In fact, the junta that rules Burma has been either directly or indirectly supporting heroin production, trafficking, and money laundering in Burma with the help of such transnational corporations as the Pepsi Cola Company. These transnational companies can make very good financial deals with the military government if they are willing to disregard world opinion about their willingness to work with the junta. The Free Burma Coalition in the United States led a boycott against the Pepsi Cola Company to try to stop Pepsi Cola from investing in and building Pizza Huts and Kentucky Fried Chicken restaurants in Burma. As a result, the Pepsi Cola Company issued the following statement: "Based on our assessment of the spirit of current US government foreign policy, we are completing our total disengagement from the Burmese market. Accordingly, we have severed all relationships with our former franchise bottler, effective January 15, 1997" (Free Burma Coalition, 2000).

Furthermore, without the precursor chemicals needed to make heroin, heroin could not be made. Acetic anhydride, an essential chemical in the production of heroin, and ephedrine, the principal chemical ingredient of methamphetamine, are imported into Burma primarily from China (Central Intelligence Agency, 2000).

Burma's Drug Problem

Until 1988 there was no discernible heroin problem in Burma. However, between 1988 and 1998, heroin use became widespread in Burma. Before 1988 there were few heroin addicts, although a sizable population of traditional people smoked opium (common among some ethnic groups). Opium use has continued to be stable at about 120,000 users over the last twenty years; heroin use has increased from nearly no heroin addicts in 1988 to 300,000 in 1998. Compared to the United States with 600,000 heroin addicts (0.002 percent of the total U.S. population), Burma has half as many heroin addicts (300,000) (over 0.007 percent of the total Burmese population) (Bureau for International Narcotics and Law Enforcement Affairs, 1999).

Documentation indicates that the production of opium doubled one year after the creation of the State Law and Order Restoration Council (SLORC), which represented the military junta that ruled Burma at the beginning of the twenty-first century. The heroin epidemic started shortly after the repression of millions of Burma's people who, after years of military rule, demanded democracy in a nonviolent uprising. The increase in domestic heroin use in Burma followed closely behind the junta's solidification of power. In 2000, their control of the country was nearly complete. The junta has remained in power and has expanded its control over all of Burma through a combination of brutal repression, attraction of foreign investment capital, and high levels of military spending. The one sector of the economy the junta denies involvement in is the drug industry, although opium is Burma's most lucrative cash crop and probably involves Burma's military (Southeast Asian Information Network, 1998).

Despite the junta's restrictions on foreign travel, there is overwhelming evidence that, at the end of the twentieth century, Burma was still the world's leading heroin-producing nation, although it is closely followed by Afghanistan. Burma's heroin addiction problem exploded in the last ten years of the twentieth century and so did the HIV/AIDS epidemic among intravenous drug users.

Brief Profile of Burma

Burma, officially known as the Union of Myanmar since 1989, is located east of Bangladesh and west of Laos and Thailand, in Southeast Asia. The total area is 261,218 square miles (676,552 square kilometers). The capital, largest city, and principal seaport is Yangon (formerly known as Rangoon). There is a horseshoe-shaped mountain range in the north of the country and a valley region in the middle of the country, which was created by the Irrawaddy River system. Some of the mountains in the north have an elevation of over 19,000 feet (6,300 meters). The Hkakabo Razi, the tallest mountain in the range, is located in the eastern part of the Himalayan Range. It is the highest peak in Southeast Asia. There are two other mountain ranges: the Arakan Yoma range forms a barrier between Burma and the subcontinent of India to the west, and the Bilauktaung Range borders Thailand on the east. These mountain ranges are natural barriers to the movement of heroin. Opium and heroin from Burma are transported into China around the Himalayan Range and into the countries that formerly were in the Soviet Union. The Shan Plateau is not a barrier between eastern Burma and China.

Forests cover 41 percent of Burma. Among other exotic and rare flora, Burma's forests are home to most of the world's remaining teak trees. The country also has mineral deposits including petroleum, metal ores, coal, and gemstones including jade and rubies.

The vast majority of the Burmese people are Buddhists, most of whom adhere to Theravada Buddhism. The center of life for most rural Burmese villagers is the Buddhist monastery which typically is located in the middle of the village. Almost 75 percent of the population (estimated to be 41,734,853 in the year 1998) lives in small rural villages.

In 2000 it was estimated that the life expectancy for the total Burmese population was fifty-five years. For males it was 53.6 years, and for females it was 56.29 years (*Encarta*, 1998). Life expectancy estimates for Burma must now take into account the effects of excess mortality caused by AIDS, which can result in lower life expectancy, higher infant mortality and death rates, lower population and growth rates, and changes in the distribution of population by age and sex.

Child Labor

Child labor is common in Burma. It is a part of a larger vicious circle in which a basic primary school education is denied to the majority of school-age children. This situation results in widespread poverty, but children need to work as soon as possible to help support the family. Although Burma has a compulsory education law, almost 40 percent of children never enroll in school, and only between 25 percent and 35 percent of children complete the five years of compulsory education (Karen Human Rights Group, 1997).

The SLORC closed schools several times between 1988 and 2000. Schools at all levels were closed for much of 1997 out of apparent concern that students might publicly protest or challenge government policies, as they did in October and December of 1996. In the year 2000, universities were still closed. Rangoon University, established in 1920, and Mandalay University, established in 1925, are the major institutions of higher learning but have been mostly closed since 1988 (Karen Human Rights Group, 2000).

Burma's GDP was approximately $60 billion (U.S.) in 1999. The per capita GDP was $1,200 (U.S.) in 1999. Some 25% of the population lives in poverty in Burma (Central Intelligence Agency, 2000).

The military junta keeps count on the number of Burmese available to serve in the military. In 1999, 11,866,000 males between the ages of fifteen and forty-nine were available for military service; 11,895,000 females between these ages were also available for military service. In Burma, both sexes can be required to serve in the military. As much as $40 million (U.S.) was spent on the Burmese military in fiscal year 1997/1998 (Central Intelligence Agency, 2000).

The Burmese government has been seeking foreign investment to help its battered narco-economy. Reluctantly, however, because of the loss of access to Burma's natural resources, most countries and businesses around the world have boycotted trade with Burma because of its poor record on human rights and its failure to reduce heroin production and trafficking across its borders.

VIGNETTE

"Are we still in Thailand, or have we crossed into Burma?," asked one of the Thai soldiers. The question was not a joke. When the small military Thai unit arrived at the remote villages along the Thai-Burmese border in Chiang

Mai, the people of the village looked different from most Thai people. The language they spoke was a version of Burmese; the houses they built had a peculiar design not typical of Thailand. The Thai Third Army was stepping up its efforts to "stabilize" border areas in the north. The border area between Burma and Thailand was very sensitive because, on the other side of the border, territory belonging to Burma was under the control of a Burmese drug lord who was also the leader of a minority insurgency group.

The primary objective of the Thai military effort was to win the hearts of the people living in the border areas with Burma. "We don't know who's who any more," said Lieutenant General Sommai Vichavorn, commander of the Third Army, when asked about the settlement on the Thai side of the border in relation to Burma's ethnic minority groups. "In some villages, we found there wasn't one single Thai villager," he said. The United Wa State Army (UWSA), the biggest drug-trafficking organization in the Golden Triangle, like other drug-trafficking minority groups before it, invested heavily in establishing an elaborate network of traffickers in Chiang Mai and Chiang Rai, two provinces in Thailand. The UWSA bought off officials and community leaders. Those who could not be paid off were driven away or killed.

The UWSA proved to be more farsighted than previous insurgency groups. They systematically placed thousands of soldiers into Thai villages to settle down with families, serve as their popular base in Thailand, and provide intelligence and materials to carry on their war. Ban Santisuk village in the Mae Chan district of Chiang Rai was almost empty during a high-profile antidrug operation; only a few had identity papers. The community had become a Wa village over the past two or three years. Some blame Thailand's own policies, which give a semblance of special treatment for ethnic minorities but have marginalized them and ensured they are second-class citizens, as well as official corruption. "It's impossible that old settlers [with legal papers] do not accommodate one way or another new settlers, it's impossible that local officials don't know," Vichavorn said. "The Wa can integrate easily because they speak Chinese." Most of the settlers along the Thai-Burmese border are Chinese-speaking families of former soldiers of the Chinese Nationalist Army, which were used by the Thai government to fight against Thai Communist insurgents in the difficult mountainous areas in the north. Most of these Chinese expatriates were strategically located as buffers to help guard the northern frontier against Burma. Additionally, other government agencies help build roads and irrigation networks. Colonel Sawasdi Krataithong, who has been overseeing the project since 1994, said it was important to take a moderate approach to Burmese villagers who live in these border villages. "Not all of the Burmese are infiltrators from drug organizations; there are many ordinary villagers who look hopefully to Thailand for sanctuary" (Khuenkaew and Chiang Rai, 1999).

SUBSTANCE ABUSE IN BURMA AND BASIC DEMOGRAPHICS

Opium production has doubled since 1988 to 4,000 metric tons a year—10 tons of opium yield one ton of heroin. Most of the opium is produced in Southeast Asia's "Golden Triangle," which spans the borders of Thailand, Burma, and Laos. The Golden Triangle became famous during the Vietnam War when the Central Intelligence Agency smuggled opium out of the Golden Triangle to help pay for its clandestine operations in Southeast Asia (Central Intelligence Agency, 2000).

Burma has been one of the world's largest producers of opium since 1988. The 1997 yield was 7,900 metric tons (Bureau for International Narcotics and Law Enforcement Affairs, 1999). The rise in opium production occurred after the takeover in Burma by the current military junta.

Heroin is a global threat. The United States has 600,000 heroin addicts—2 percent of the world's total population of heroin addicts. Europe has some 1.5 million heroin addicts; Pakistan, 2 million heroin addicts; and Thailand, 600,000 addicts. China, India, and Iran report a growing heroin problem.

Burma has long been the prime source of heroin for the United States and for the world market. Afghanistan now threatens to overtake Burma in production volume, and Nigerian heroin traffickers have created a highly developed worldwide network of heroin wholesalers. Cultivation usually takes place in inaccessible growing areas. Proceeds from retail heroin sales may be nearly $10 billion in the United States and $25 billion in Europe (McCaffrey, 1996).

Use and Purity of Heroin

Combinations of heroin and crack cocaine, which are smoked, were used in New York by 2000. The negative impact of long-term crack use led many drug abusers to use heroin to soften the impact of crack. Smoking became the preferred method of using heroin because it was available in a form pure enough to smoke. There is a strong relationship between how heroin is used and its purity and physical properties (whether it is Mexican brown, black tar, or white powder). For example, when heroin is in the form of white powder and has high purity, the user can achieve the desired effects through snorting or smoking. It takes less heroin to reach the same high when the heroin is injected. Chronic heroin addicts typically inject heroin. Extremely pure heroin is now available at low prices. Toward the end of 1999, in northern Burma, high-grade heroin cost approximately $175 per kilo (Central Intelligence Agency, 2000).

Low prices means increased health problems related to drug abuse and drug overdose. The minimum lethal dose of heroin is 200 milligrams, although people who have developed a tolerance can survive higher doses.

Mixing heroin with other drugs can result in a deadly cocktail. Taking heroin (100 milligrams) intravenously with alcohol and/or barbiturates or cocaine will result in coma and death. These combinations of alcohol and heroin, barbiturate and heroin, and cocaine and heroin account for hundreds of deaths a year.

Rising Flood of Opium

In East Asia, governments have increasingly become alarmed about the growing threat to their societies posed by the rising flood of opium pouring out of Burma and Afghanistan. China faces a serious and growing domestic drug abuse problem in its provinces along its border with Burma and in the provinces that serve as a major route for heroin trafficking across the land to Eastern Europe.

No one really knows how large the Burmese heroin industry is, but there are some excellent estimates based on different sources involved in the heroin trade. A 1984 estimate of the value of the heroin trade along Burma's borders was $500 million (U.S.). This increased to $850 million (U.S.) in 1995 and was over $1.2 billion in 1997. In 1999 there was a serious drought in the opium-growing areas of Burma. As a result, opium production dropped from approximately 2,900 metric tons to 1,100 metric tons—a 38 percent drop. Between 1995 and 1998, opium cultivation grew by 6 percent, and heroin production increased by 9 percent. In the fiscal year 1995/1996, 163,100 hectares of poppy were cultivated. That amount of poppy can produce 2,560 metric tons of opium or 197 metric tons of heroin (Tasker and Crispin, 2000; U.S. State Department, 1999). Plainly, opium, heroin, and amphetamines are among Burma's largest exports and of great benefit to the military junta. With sharp increases in military spending, and severe shortages of foreign capital to make purchases on the world market for goods and services that cannot be produced in Burma, narco money is the only source of income. Heroin exporting and money laundering are semilegitimate businesses and investments in Burma which have the knowledge and unofficial support of the junta.

HISTORY OF ALCOHOL AND DRUG USE IN BURMA

Burma has a long history of migration and conflict among its various ethnic groups. Fixed borders were not delineated until the British Imperial government in Burma established them in the 1820s. Under British control, diverse peoples far from Rangoon were governed by a central administration. Despite the efforts of the British, many remote areas effectively maintained self-rule throughout their regime. During World War II, many Burmese joined the Japanese forces, but many minority ethnic groups remained loyal to the British. This reflected a genuine desire for independence on the part of both groups: the Burmese wanted to be free of the British colonial yoke, and ethnic minorities wished to escape the domination of the Burmese ethnic groups over them (Open Society Institute, 2000).

Burma became the Union of Burma and gained independence in 1948. Extensive negotiations led by General Aung San convinced most ethnic minority groups to join the new union. The Panglong Agreement of 1947 outlined minority rights and specifically gave the Shan and Karenni peoples the option to secede from the union a decade after independence. Almost immediately after gaining independence, Burma was drawn into a series of brutal ethnic wars that continued throughout the last half of the twentieth century and into the twenty-first century (Open Society Institute, 2000).

After receiving its independence from Britain in 1948, Burma was run by an elected government until 1958 when a military coup d'état overthrew the government. Apart from a brief return to democracy between 1960 and 1962, Burma has been ruled by a military government since 1958 (International Labor Affairs, 1998).

In 1988 students, workers, Buddhist monks, and even members of the armed services took part in a pro-democracy demonstration to protest the economic and political conditions imposed by the military junta. Reports indicate that thousands of protesters were killed and injured by the junta's armed forces when they attacked demonstrators to put a stop to the peaceful demonstrations. The repercussions from around the world to their violent actions forced the junta to form a new military governing body to rule the country. This group took the name the State Law and Order Restoration Council (SLORC) and imposed martial law on the country (Karen Human Rights Group, 1997).

In 1997 the SLORC renamed itself the State Peace and Development Council (SPDC), although the military presence and repressive policies remained essentially the same. The regime still refuses to transfer power to the legitimate, elected government and remains a nondemocratic, military dictatorship (International Labor Affairs, 1998).

In 1999 the SPDC conducted free elections after declaring its intention to transfer power to a civilian government. Many opposition politicians, however, were arrested and detained before the election. Even so, the National League for Democracy (NLD), the opposition party, won 80 percent of the seats for a new legislative body. Disappointed in the results of the vote, the SPDC did not honor its promise to turn the government over to the election winners (Karen Human Rights Group, 2000).

More Than Fifty Years of Ethnic Wars

There is no reliable census data that can be used to estimate the composition of Burma's ethnic mosaic. It is assumed that population data in Burma is skewed to exaggerate the number of people who belong to the

Burman ethnic group. At any rate, the best estimates are that among the ethnic Burmese groups, the largest ethnic group is Burman, which makes up about 33 percent of Burma's approximately 42 million people. The Burman ethnic group controls the army and the government. Most of Burma's other ethnic minorities inhabit the mountainous frontiers. The Karen and Shan groups each represent about 10 percent of the population; the Akha, Chin, Chinese, Danu, Indian, Kachin, Karenni, Kayan, Kokang, Lahu, Mon, Naga, Palaung, Pao, Rakhine, Rohingya, Tavoyan, and Wa peoples each constitute 5 percent or less of the population. The Wa people of Burma are of special interest to the issue of worldwide substance abuse. The Wa have been cultivating opium poppies for centuries, but in recent years production has increased so dramatically that Wa opium production has become one of the largest in the world cultivated by one group. Wa opium accounts for about 80 percent of the opium shipped out of Burma.

The ethnic wars in Burma started over demands made by Burma's ethnic minorities for genuine autonomy in their home areas and for the legal right to participate in the affairs of Burma as a whole. The often bloody wars between the junta's government troops and the ethnic armies have been responsible for thousands of displaced people and refugees. For instance, in 1991, the Rohingya people (for the most part Muslim) in southeastern Burma were attacked by the junta's government troops, and more than 250,000 Rohingya people fled to neighboring Bangladesh. In another case, at least 110,000 Karen and Mon people from eastern Burma became refugees in Thailand following a deadly Burmese army offensive in 1994 (Khuenkaew and Chiang Rai, 1999).

One of the first cease-fires to be held involved the Wa and Kokang armies, which until 1987 were a part of the Burmese Communist Party. The Burmese government's agreements with these two groups gave them permission to cultivate and trade opium without interference from the Burmese government. This resulted in a sharp increase in opium and heroin production and smuggling from Burma. A worldwide rise in heroin use and addiction followed (Khuenkaew and Chiang Rai, 1999).

SUBSTANCE ABUSE IN BURMA TODAY

Political Views and Public Policies

Basic elements of the rule of law were never recognized by the military junta. Moreover, despite the tradition of British law, military rulers in Burma have disregarded the rule of law since they took power in the 1960s. Even more discouraging for the Burmese people, the few vestiges of constitutional government and legal authority that did exist at the time of the coup have all but disappeared (Soberano, 1999). At the end of the millennium, there was no legislative body composed of elected representatives. Members of the executive branch were not elected, and the judiciary was not independent of the executive branch of the government. The SLORC suspended both the 1947 and the 1974 constitutions. The military governments of Burma have continually denied access to vital information related to the politically sensitive issue of human rights (International Labor Affairs, 1998).

Political Ramifications of the Heroin Trade

Until lasting political solutions are found in Burma, the struggle of democracy movements and the wars for the rights of ethnic minority groups will continue. Certainly, under these conditions, drug addiction and HIV./AIDS will continue to devastate the Burmese in the opium-growing areas. The involvement of the junta in the heroin trade has been a tragedy in the history of Burma in many ways. The junta involvement in the heroin trade has blighted the country's reputation, and the junta can certainly be implicated in making heroin widely available and cheap to the Burmese people. These and other infrastructure problems make it all the more difficult to establish drug prevention and treatment programs, as well as HIV/AIDS prevention and treatment programs (Soberano, 1999).

Consequences of Addiction

The heroin HIV/AIDS highway from hell runs between Chittagong in Burma, into China through Chengdu, from Almaty into the southeastern area of the Gobi Desert, and into the underbelly of Eastern Europe. The Burmese government estimated that in 1994 as many as 1 percent of adult men nationwide were active injecting drug users, higher in the drug-producing areas. A United Nations report estimated that, in early 1994, between 60 and 70 percent of all injecting drug users in Burma had HIV. The figures for specific cities included 74 percent in Yongon (Rangoon), 84 percent in Mandalay, and 91 percent in Myitkyina, the capital of the Kachin State on the Burma-China border (Department of Health, Yangon, 1997).

There is no doubt that the high rates of HIV infection among injecting drug users in Burma is caused by needle sharing. In Burma, it is currently illegal to possess syringes, except for medical purposes. Syringes are in extremely short supply, making needle sharing a daily reality among Burma's heroin addicts. In the poor areas, "professional injectors" work in "tea stalls" (shooting galleries) where they re-use needles to inject heroin addicts. These tea stalls are major sources of HIV transmission. In remote areas of Burma, addicts often make their own crude injecting equipment; sharing further promotes the spread of the HIV infection (Southeast Asian Information Network, 1998).

Needle sharing is also known to spread hepatitis B and C viruses, syphilis, malaria, and tetanus. A Japanese group in the late 1990s reported the prevalence of HIV and hepatitis viruses among injecting drug users, patients with sexually transmitted diseases, sex workers, and others in Burma. They found that among 531 persons who were HIV positive, 12 percent also had an acute hepatitis B infection, and 40 percent of the group had a previous hepatitis B infection. Among the 291 subjects who were injecting drug users, 98 percent had an HIV infection. The only conclusion that can be drawn from these numbers is that needle sharing is a common practice among the Burmese who inject drugs (Southeast Asian Information Network, 1998).

A qualitative study conducted among 3,200 high-risk Burmese (drug users, truckers, miners, and sex workers) found that many past opium smokers had switched to heroin injection owing to the lower cost of heroin. The study also reported that opium smokers were more likely to employ a sex worker than drug injectors. Condom use with sex workers was rare. No addicts interviewed reported sterilizing needles; needle sharing was extremely common; and knowledge of HIV/AIDS was "very low" (Southeast Asian Information Network, 1998).

One thing is clear, there is widespread fear, among those who are AIDS/HIV infected, of the junta government and its policies toward infected persons. This fear is a strong deterrent to voluntary HIV/AIDS testing in Burma. There are reports of the segregation of women returning from Thailand thought to be, or known to be, HIV infected. These women have been kept in detention centers and housed in rural leprosariums in at least two districts controlled by the military government. The women in these centers fear contracting leprosy and HIV (Medicins du Mond, 1997; Southeast Asian Information Network, 1998).

The interaction of HIV and leprosy is currently unknown, but it could lead to the spread of one, or both, infections. The leprosy agent, *Mycobacterium leprae*, is closely related to *Mycobacterium tuberculosis*. The latter's interaction with HIV is well described—and deadly. Tuberculosis rates have more than doubled in most countries affected by HIV/AIDS, and tuberculosis is thought to be the most common opportunistic infection among HIV/AIDS patients in Burma (Medicins du Mond, 1997; Southeast Asian Information Network, 1998).

Drug Treatment and Rehabilitation in Burma

In Burma, drug addiction is considered both a medical and a behavioral problem which may lead an individual to pursue criminal activity. It also may further the spread and the use of illicit drugs throughout the population. Therefore, medical, social, and legislative interventions are needed to deal with drug addicts in order to help them to achieve full recovery. For these reasons, a 1974 law provides for compulsory treatment and rehabilitation of drug addicts. The Ministry of Health has set up treatment centers for detoxification and the medical rehabilitation of young drug abusers. In addition, two large comprehensive centers were established in August 1982 to provide inpatient treatment for addicts who are between sixteen and forty years of age. The primary objectives of treatment and rehabilitation at these centers are to help addicts restore their physical health, achieve psychosocial adjustment, and, through training, acquire occupational and vocational skills to obtain employment (Khant and Win, 1978; Khant, 1985).

Following detoxification, it is believed that aftercare, rehabilitation, and social reintegration are much more effective with organized community support. For these reasons, the government has mobilized the mass media to alert communities to both the problems of drug abuse and the possibilities of their effective involvement in combating drug abuse and related problems. In those communities where there are many drug addicts, detoxification services are provided at the local level. In communities with young drug experimenters, emphasis is placed on developing alternative programs to drug use such as recreational activities, leadership training programs, and voluntary labor contribution schemes. These programs are organized and carried out under the guidance of local authorities (Khant, 1985).

In Burma, registration and treatment for drug addiction are compulsory under state law. If an addict refuses to register, he or she could be sentenced to prison for a minimum of five years. As a result, over 43 percent of drug offenders are in Burmese prisons. Confidentiality, a cornerstone of treatment in many developed countries, is not a right of drug addicts in Burma. In fact, every citizen of Burma is legally required to report any drug addict with whom they come into contact. Of those registered as drug users, who were treated at Burmese drug treatment centers and hospitals between 1974 and 1994, 62.3 % used opium and 28 percent used heroin. In some Burmese states, those treated for heroin addiction was much higher. In the state of Yangon, 88.4 percent of those treated were addicted to heroin; 11.6 percent were treated for opium use. In the state of Kachin (where Burmese military control is tight but not complete), 86.1 percent were treated for heroin addiction, and 13.9 percent were treated for opium addiction (Bureau for International Narcotics and Law Enforcement Affairs, 1999). Professional treatment for heroin and opium addiction included gradual detoxification and religious therapy. Drug treatment undertaken by insurgents or rebel forces often takes the form of abrupt withdrawal to detoxify the addict and the threat of being shot if the addict refuses detoxification.

Although government statistics continue to show a relatively small number of registered opium and heroin addicts (those who check into a government-run treatment facility), government resources devoted to countering this growing domestic problem remain woefully inadequate. The entire country has only six major drug treatment centers, with a total of 220 beds, and additional outpatient facilities at twenty-four smaller centers.

The Ministry of Health has the lead responsibility for Burma's drug treatment and rehabilitation efforts, although the Ministries of Education and Information contribute to the government's reduction programs through preventive education efforts. Since 1974, government treatment centers have registered 14,893 heroin addicts, 34,453 opium addicts, and 4,640 persons addicted to other substances (U.S. State Department, 1995). However, a trend noted throughout the 1980s has been the shift from opium to heroin abuse among Burmese drug addicts. According to Burmese government statistics, some 84% of new addicts registered in 1993 were addicted to heroin versus only 20 percent in 1983 (U.S. State Department, 1995). In 1982 more comprehensive programs were instituted. Two major special treatment and rehabilitation centers were open to provide long-term treatment. Wettingan had 1,200 beds and Kathekwin 40 new beds. The program consisted of detoxification and long-term rehabilitation for up to forty-two weeks (Khant, 1985).

Because treatment of drug addiction remains rudimentary and focuses on prosecution, prisons have shockingly high rates of both drug addiction and HIV. Drug treatment services are not reaching most drug users because of a lack of facilities and a lack of adequately trained personnel. Addiction and the spread of HIV/AIDS have become cross-border problems of concern to China as well, particularly in Yunnan Province, on Burma's northern border (U.S. State Department, 1995).

Social Views, Customs, and Practices

The social fabric of Burma has been ripped apart by a military-led government which has used strategies rejected by democratic nations to retain power. Heroin, the government's tool for generating income and for breaking the will of its people, continues to scar the Burmese consciousness as it does their bodies. At the beginning of the millennium, Burma faced the problems of continued ethnic war, addiction, HIV/AIDS, forced labor, refugees, and an infrastructure so chaotic that it cannot support a stable population or the programming needed to regenerate itself. This has left vulnerable groups without protection from those who would exploit them. When the Burmese people are exploited by international firms, kickbacks generally benefit the government officials.

Forced Child Labor and Child Trafficking

Burmese children have been forced to work in all areas of the economy, including as road builders, porters, sentries, and used to provide services for the military. Reports indicate the existence of child soldiers, some of them conscripts, in both the Burmese military and in the minority ethnic armed opposition groups. Former soldiers who joined the army as children reported that it was easy for boys as young as 14 to join as long as they gave their age as 18. Other child soldiers reported being ordered to beat and kill porters who could not work and to execute villagers who were suspected of collaborating with enemy troops. These child soldiers are often given amphetamines, tranquilizers, and alcohol before going into battle.

Trafficking in sex workers, or the selling of girls and children into the commercial sex industry, is one of Burma's major businesses. There are numerous reports of trafficking of children from Burma to Thailand. Some trafficked children become beggars and hawkers. The vast majority, however, are sold for the sex market. Burmese children make up the majority of the estimated 60,000 illegal workers in the Thai commercial sex industry (Thein Myint Thu, Than Swe, Bo Kywe, et al., 1995).

A Crisis Faced by Youth

The youth of Burma, at the beginning of the twenty-first century, are facing a crisis that will change their destiny as a generation. Most youth in Burma are barred from obtaining a fundamental education because the education system has been closed to prevent student democracy demonstrations. Many have been forced to leave the country or turn to the sex and drug trades to make enough money to survive.

Students who could be admitted to a university forfeit their education when they refuse to promise not to become involved in political activity. More fundamentally, increasing poverty has put a university education out of the reach of most young people whose families are no longer able to support them. About 300,000 students who left high school between 1996 and 2000 lost their chance for a university education for these reasons (Karen Human Rights Group, 2000). Although some universities have reopened, these "reopened" institutions have insufficient accommodation, little teaching equipment, and few trained teachers. The government's efforts to keep young Burmese out of the educational system leaves them with few marketable skills and little hope for the future. This crisis has forced many young people to turn to the sex industry, where they become alcohol dependent and drug dependent and contract HIV/AIDS (Karen Human Rights Group, 2000).

The crisis faced by young people in Burma today is the result of the junta government's oppressive policies and practices which are aimed at young people whom the junta regards as a threat to their hold on power. Although Burma's military government claims education is a priority, in the year 2000 it spent only 0.5 percent of the country's GNP on education (other Southeast Asian countries spent about 2.7 percent of their GDPs) (Karen Human Rights Group, 2000).

The Burmese Army and Heroin Production

Testimony from drug dealers, carriers, and drug users in Burma consistently implicates the junta as a major player in opium cultivation, heroin production, and distribution to the international illegal drug market. The military conflict in the Shan State was often cited by the military junta as a cause for Burma's inability to control the heroin problem; however, the ethnic groups that have signed cease-fire agreements, notably the Kachin Independence Organization (KIO), have reported that heroin use increased dramatically among their young people after the cease-fire was signed and the army took control of the Kachin State borders. This situation, tragically, has led to extremely high rates of HIV infection in Kachin State and in neighboring Yunnan Province in China (Southeast Asian Information Network, 1998).

Pacification Programs

Since 1990 almost all of the minority ethnic groups of Burma have signed a cease-fire agreement with the junta, with the notable exception of the Karen National Union (KNU) and the Chin National Front (CNF). As part of these cease-fire agreements, the SPDC promised education, health, and development investments organized out of the Border Areas Development Program (BAD). The BAD programs, however, never delivered on the promised investments. The recent decline in the Burmese economy, in the late 1990s, and the devaluation of the kyat (Burmese currency: 6.27 kyat = $1 U.S.) have further stalled progress. At an August 1996 seminar on HIV/AIDS programs, which included representatives from twenty-five Burmese ethnic groups, including the KNU and all of the major cease-fire parties, there was unanimous agreement that the BAD programs had done nothing to address either the HIV/AIDS crisis or the heroin epidemic among ethnic minority Burmans. The ethnic groups that had signed cease-fire agreements were prohibited from seeking outside funding for such help in the agreement with the junta (Khuenkaew and Chiang Rai, 1999).

The many border regions of Burma, including a number of areas not under SPDC control and in conflict with the Burmese army, have not been studied in terms of HIV, with the exception of the Shan State areas under government control and Kachin State; both regions had severe HIV epidemics.

Burmese Refugees

The estimated number of displaced Burmans within Burma as a result of junta military action ranged from 500,000 to 1 million in 1999, although some sources put the figure at closer to 2 million (U.S. Committee for Refugees, 2000). Ethnic minorities, many of whom are rural people, constitute most of Burma's internally displaced people. However, a significant number of the majority ethnic group (the Burmans) have also been driven from their cities and villages. By and large, the displacement of these Burmese has resulted from the junta's two-prong strategy to control the ethnic minority and democracy groups: forced labor and forced relocation.

For instance, in Central Shan State, between 1996 and 1998, the Burmese military ordered more than 300,000 people to move into strategic relocation sites. During the same period, more than 80,000 Shan fled to Thailand. At the same time (in 1999), more Burmese refugees sought asylum in neighboring countries: 145,000 in Thailand (mostly ethnic minorities, along with some pro-democracy activists); 40,000 in India (mostly Chin); and 53,000 in Bangladesh (52,000 Rohingya and 1,000 Chin) (U.S. Committee for Refugees, 2000).

THE FUTURE OF SUBSTANCE ABUSE IN BURMA

The junta's continuing engagement in the drug trade, while ignoring the economic needs of the ethnic minorities in Burma, will increase the dependency of local leaders on revenues from the heroin trade. This will further undermine the ability of local minority ethnic leaders to represent their people, and this dependency will give drug traffickers a primary role in the economies of these ethnic regions. While the Kachin, Wa, and Shan people face devastating heroin and amphetamine epidemics, as well as HIV/AIDS among their young people, their chances for any valid participatory role in their country's future are being lost.

Proposed Solutions and Strategies

A peaceful, democratic, and drug-free Burma can be realized only if the concerns and grievances of the country's minority ethnic groups are addressed. Burma's democratic opposition has proposed programs to redress these problems and to achieve ethnic reconciliation and cooperation, but it will be a formidable task for any future Burmese government.

Programs to restart the economy and to open schools and universities must occur simultaneously with programs in the rural areas, such as crop substitution programs, to reduce the dependency on opium cultivation. Prevention and treatment programs to reduce drug consumption and to prevent and treat HIV/AIDS must be a part of any revitalization plan for Burma.

The substance abuse problem, the problems with the economy, and many of the problems involving minority ethnic communities are the result of the military junta's strategies to retain power. Until the junta is replaced by a government that cares for all Burmese people, the increase in heroin addiction, the increase in death from AIDS, and the continued killing in wars will go on unabated.

CONCLUSION

It is hard to imagine how an exotic land with such beautiful people as the Burmese became one of the world's largest dope dealers. Although there have been border wars for centuries and many of the ethnic Burmans have used opium for at least a thousand years without significant problems, heroin, which came on the scene in 1989, has caused devastating problems both directly in terms of mass addiction and indirectly as HIV/AIDS. The Burmese people have never suffered from invaders—neither the British during colonialism nor the Japanese during World War II—as they have suffered at the hands of the military junta, the invasion of heroin, and the HIV/AIDS virus.

As the world community's drug dealer, Burma as a nation has lost its dignity and all respect from other nations of the world, and the family (the Burmese people) are the ones who suffer the most.

If the demand for heroin were not so great in the developed countries of the world and if drug addicts in the incredibly lucrative American illegal drug market were not willing to pay such high prices for heroin, the international illegal drug cartels and the military junta in Burma would not use their resources to cultivate poppies and manufacture heroin. Even without the military junta, peace and democracy in Burma will require a harmonious accommodation among the country's diverse ethnic groups. Without lasting resolution to questions of local autonomy and national power sharing, rebellions that have flared and simmered in Burma's borderlands for nearly five decades cannot be resolved. Without peace, there is little chance for a grassroots economic development that could reduce opium production and heroin trafficking in many impoverished areas of Burma.

REFERENCES

Agence France Presse. (1996, November 28). *Opium production increasing dramatically—report*. Paris, France: Author.

Bureau for International Narcotics and Law Enforcement Affairs. (1999). *International narcotics control strategy report: Burma statistics tables*. Washington, DC: U.S. State Department.

Burma Department of Health. (1996). *Disease control programme*. Myanmar: Yangon.

———. (1997). *Annual report of the AIDS prevention and control programme*. Myanmar: Yangon.

Central Intelligence Agency. (2000). *The world factbook: Burma*. Washington, DC: prepared by the Central Intelligence Agency for the use of U.S. government officials. Retrieved November 12, 2000, from the World Wide Web: http://www.odci.gov/cia/publications/factbook/geos/fr.htm

Department of Health, Yangon. (1997). *Annual report of the AIDS prevention and control programme, Myanmar 1996.* Yangon, Myanmar: Disease Control Programme, Department of Health, Yangon.

Encarta Desk Encyclopedia (1998). Microsoft Corporation, CD-ROM.

Free Burma Coalition (2000). *PepsiCo/Burmese human rights abuse.* Washington, DC: Author. Retrieved November 12, 2000, from the World Wide Web: http://www.ibiblio.org/freeburma/

International Labor Affairs. (1998). *Report on labor practices in Burma.* Washington, DC: U.S. State Department.

Karen Human Rights Group. (1997). *Forced labor: Submission to the ILO.* San Francisco: Karen National League. Retrieved November 15, 2000, from the World Wide Web: www.karen.org/

————. (2000). *Education crisis forces Burma youth into sex, drugs trade: activists.* San Francisco: Karen National League. Retrieved November 15, 2000, from the World Wide Web: www.karen.org/news/

Khant, U. (1985). *Compulsory treatment and rehabilitation programmes.* Geneva, Switzerland: United Nations International Drug Control Programme.

Khant, U., and Win, N. (1978). *Drug abuse in the Socialist Republic of the Union of Burma.* National Institute on Drug Abuse, Research Monograph Series no. 19. Washington, DC: U.S. Government Printing Office.

Khuenkaew, Subin, and Chiang Rai, Nusara Thaitawat (1999, August 16). Drug suppression: Soldiers try to win ethnic hearts at border. *Bangkok Post,* (Thailand), p. 1A.

McCaffrey, B. (1996, September 19). *Heroin: A global threat.* Washington, DC: Federal News Service.

Medicins du Mond. (1997, October). *Sexual and drug behaviour, knowledge, and attitudes about AIDS in Myanmar targeted populations.* Paper presented at the Fourth International Conference on AIDS in Asia and the Pacific, Manila, Philippines.

Open Society Institute. (2000). *The Burma project: Ethnic groups.* The Burma Project of the Open Society Institute, Washington DC: Author. Retrieved November 12, 2000, from the World Wide Web: http://www.soros.org/burma/welcome.html

Soberano, R.G. (1999). *Burma: Role of drugs in power grab.* Phoenix: Asian Chamber of Commerce.

Southeast Asian Information Network. (1998). *Out of Control 2: The HIV/AIDS epidemic in Burma.* Southeast Asian Information Network. Retrieved November 14, 2000, from the World Wide Web: http://www.ibiblio.org/freeburma/drugs/ooc2/

Tasker, R. and Crispin, S.W. (2000). *Frustration over Burma's illegal trade is reaching dangerous levels in Thailand.* San Francisco: Karen National League. Retrieved November 15, 2000, from the World Wide Web: www.karen.org/news/

Thein Myint Thu, Than Swe, Bo Kywe, et al. (1995, September 17–21). "Sexual Risk Behaviours in Young Soldiers HIV & VDRL Seroprevalence," Department of Defense Medical Services, Myanmar, Abstract B304, the 111 International Conference on AIDS in Asia and the Pacific, Chiangmai, Thailand.

U.S. Committee for Refugees. (2000). *Country report: Burma*. Washington, DC: U.S. Author.

U.S. State Department. (1995). *International narcotics control strategy report*. Washington, DC: Bureau for International Narcotics and Law Enforcement Affairs.

———. (1999). *International narcotics control strategy report*. Washington, DC: Bureau for International Narcotics and Law Enforcement Affairs.

Yoshihara, N., Matsuo, M., and Takebe, Y. (1997). *High incidence of viral hepatitis among HIV seropositive persons in Myanmar*. Paper presented at the Fourth International Conference on AIDS in Asia and the Pacific, Manila, Philippines.

2

CANADA

Douglas Rugh

INTRODUCTION

Canada is influenced by both the United States and its European heritage. Because of the tension between these sometimes different points of view, Canada's policies appear to be at a crossroads between the prohibition/criminalization and the harm-reduction methods of dealing with their own domestic drug problem. The government states in official documents that its overall policy objective includes the desire to reduce the harm done by drugs and alcohol to society. However, strict punishment for possession and the large amount of funding spent on the punitive system raise the question of which is doing more harm—the policies enacted to fight drug abuse or the drugs themselves. This chapter examines both the prohibition/criminalization and harm-reduction policies.

Brief Profile of Canada

Canada, with a total area of 9,970,610 square kilometers (3,849,674 square miles), is the world's second largest country after Russia. This vast country has a relatively small population, which is concentrated along the southern border. Canada is located in the northern latitudes, and consequently cold weather influences the society. Approximately 77 percent of all Canadians are urban dwellers, and approximately three-quarters of them inhabit a narrow belt along the border with the United States.

The population of Canada is 30,337,334 (1997 estimate). In Canada, 35 percent are of British origin; 25 percent, French; 20 percent, other European descent; 10 percent, Asian; 3 percent, indigenous Indians or Inuits; and 7 percent, other. Both English and French are official languages of Canada (60 percent speak English as the primary language, 24 percent speak French); Native American languages and the Inuit language, Inuktitut, are also spoken. The labor force consists of 15,726,000 with a 1995 unemployment rate of 9.5 percent. Roman Catholics make up the largest religious group in Canada; nearly half of them are found in Québec. The largest Protestant denomination is the United Church of Canada, followed by the Anglican Church of Canada. About one-eighth of Canadians claim to have no religion. (Reed and Hiebert, 2000).

The head of state in Canada is the British monarch. The official head of government is the governor-general, who is appointed by the monarch on the recommendation of Canada's prime minister. The governor-general follows the advice of the majority in the House of Commons in appointing the prime minister, who is the effective head of government.

The Canadian economy depends heavily on agriculture. Canada is a leading exporter of food products. Wheat is the most important crop, and Canada annually produces more than one-fifth of the world's supply. Livestock accounts for half of yearly farm income. Cattle ranching prevails in the west. Forest products provide a significant portion of Canadian exports, and Canada leads the world in newsprint production. Canada is a major exporter of fishing products and is a world leader in mineral exports, including crude petroleum, natural gas, metals, and coal.

The gross domestic product (GDP) in 1996 was U.S.$579 billion, or U.S.$19,330 per person. In 1994 the military consumed 5.81 percent of the national GDP. In the same year, the active troop strength was 70,500. There are 912,200 kilometers (566,830 miles) of roads in Canada and 440 passenger vehicles per 1,000 persons. There are eleven international airports. There are 714 television sets and 1,053 radios for each 1,000 persons. The life expectancy at birth in Canada in 1997 was seventy-six years of age for males and eighty-two years of age for females. There is one hospital bed for every 196 people and one physician for every 455 persons. Infant mortality is 7 per 1,000 live births, but it is much higher for some minority groups and the poor.

Elementary and secondary education is free and compulsory. The duration of compulsory education is ten years between the ages of six and sixteen. Approximately 97 percent of the people in Canada are officially literate.

VIGNETTE

The following is an example of a woman speaking at an AA meeting.
"My name is Lisa and I am an alcoholic.
"The disease of alcoholism knows no age limit. I picked up my first top-

shelf drink at the age of thirty-two and proceeded to drink for twenty-five years."

Lisa said she did not know that every drink was leading her to alcoholism. She had ten years as a social drinker, then ten years as a binge drinker.

"From then on there was not a day without a drink, without a blackout, without the compulsion to drink.

"I knew I had a problem, a sinking feeling that everything was getting out of control, but I did not know that it was alcoholism."

Her sister suggested she contact a mutual friend who was a member of Alcoholics Anonymous.

She contacted AA and two women came to see her. That Wednesday night she attended her first AA meeting.

"I had quite a lot of liquor in me, and for three months I continued to drink before and after meetings."

Asked if she could manage one day of sobriety and then another, Lisa managed to last twenty days before she bought another bottle.

"I drank for seven days from dawn to dusk. I slept where I fell. I woke up bruised, not knowing how I got the bruises. I was crying inside but did not know how to stop.

"It was 6 A.M. and I decided that I would hang myself."

She tidied up, cleaned and showered, still drinking, and went into the garage. She put a rope over a roof beam, stood on a stool, and put the rope around her neck.

Then she hesitated. "I said, 'God help me, what am I doing.' "

She came down from the stool and rang AA again. It was suggested she go to a treatment center.

"I agreed but continued to drink all that day.

"It was a terrible time: the remorse, the crying, not being able to control the drink.

"With one day's sobriety I was full of grief; lonely, depressed, and resentful; possessing little help.

"To me alcoholics were drunks, the ones we saw on the side of the road. It took me a long time to realize that I too was an alcoholic.

"All of a sudden I knew. I burst into tears and ran from the room. Then I knew we all had a common bond and realized that this was the beginning of recovery.

"The program cleansed me spiritually, gave me strength and hope, and returned my will to live.

"I am truly thankful to God for giving me another chance."

OVERVIEW OF SUBSTANCE ABUSE IN CANADA

It is commonly thought among social scientists that Canada's indigenous people did not use alcohol because the climate is not conducive to its production. Some scientists go so far as to say that Canada's indigenous people did not use any psychoactive substances before the arrival of the Europeans (Smart, 1983). If this is true, this population is unique because throughout history societies everywhere have produced and used various drugs and alcohol.

According to the Canadian Center on Substance Abuse, the declining trend in alcohol sales observed throughout the 1980s and 1990s did not continue in 1996–1997. Sales, in terms of alcohol content, increased from 7.4 liters (almost 2 gallons) per person in 1995–1996 to 7.6 liters (2 gallons) per person in 1996–1997, the first increase to occur since the early 1980s.

It is estimated that 6,504 Canadians (4,681 men and 1,823 women) lost their lives as a result of alcohol consumption in 1995, and 80,946 were hospitalized (51,765 men and 29,181 women) due to alcohol in 1995–1996. Motor vehicle accidents, liver cirrhosis, and suicide accounted for the largest number of alcohol-related deaths, while accidental falls, alcohol dependence syndrome, and motor vehicle accidents accounted for the largest number of alcohol-related hospitalizations. In 1995, 803 deaths (695 men and 108 women) in Canada were attributed to illicit drugs. Suicides (329 deaths) and opiate poisoning (160 deaths) accounted for almost two-thirds of all drug-related deaths. The 803 deaths resulted in 33,669 potential years of life lost. In 1995–1996, 6,947 hospitalizations were attributed to illicit drugs (Single et al., 1996).

Policy to Deal with Drug and Alcohol Addiction

An increase in illicit drug use in the 1960s and the 1970s was met by greatly increased criminalization. Despite the high individual and social costs, the prohibition of illicit drug possession with penalties of up to seven years of imprisonment appears to have had relatively little deterrent effect. Rates of use climbed sharply through the 1960s and early 1970s, despite the large allocation of enforcement resources. The strain on the courts, and the rising numbers of otherwise law-abiding youth being sentenced for drug offenses (particularly cannabis possession), created pressure for the liberalization of Canada's drug laws.

The Commission of Inquiry in the Non-Medical Use of Drugs (referred to as the Le Dain Commission) was formed in 1969 to address this growing concern about drug use and appropriate responses. The Le Dain Commission described and analyzed the social costs and individual consequences of the criminalization policy (Riley, 1998).

The Le Dain Commission identified the need for sweeping police powers as a social cost of drug policy. Under special provisions, a law enforcement officer in Canada has broader powers of search and seizure—in even minor drug cases—than he has in a murder, rape, or other serious criminal case.

Some enforcement methods associated with drug investigations contradict personal rights and freedoms. Wiretaps, paid informants, undercover agents, police dogs, arrests without warning, surprise raids, strip searches, and the granting of immunity to suspects in return for information are all legal procedures. Such methods have been widely criticized for impugning the integrity of the police and the criminal justice system, particularly among youth. These powers have been expanded under the new drug law to include what is called a "reverse sting," in which a police officer can legally sell drugs to a buyer in order to have grounds for arrest (Riley, 1998).

Following much consultation and further study, the still active Le Dain Commission concluded that drug prohibition results in high costs but relatively little benefit. The majority of the commissioners recommended a gradual withdrawal from criminal sanctions against users, along with the development of less coercive and costly alternatives to replace the punitive application of criminal law.

Attempts to reduce the consequences of criminalization have met with limited success. A bill that would have decriminalized possession of cannabis (Bill S-19) was introduced but defeated in 1975 (Riley, 1998). Despite some attempts for balance, the dominant policy regarding illicit drugs has remained one of criminal prohibition. With the introduction of a new drug law in the 1990s, there was an opportunity to address some of the problems of past law and to benefit from what had been learned from the experience of other countries. The new law, the Controlled Drugs and Substances Act, however, is soundly prohibitionist and rather than retreating from the drug war rhetoric of the past it expands the net of prohibition even further. The problems related to criminalizing drug users, the social and economic costs of this approach, and its failure to reduce drug availability have not been addressed (Riley, 1998).

The criminal approach to drug use has several effects on drug users, health-care professionals, and society, and it may increase rather than decrease harm from drug use. Because drugs can be purchased only in the underground market, they are of unknown strength and composition, which may result in overdoses or other harm to the drug user. Fear of criminal penalties and the high price of drugs cause users to consume drugs in more efficient ways, such as by injection, which contribute to the transmission of HIV and hepatitis. Because sterile injection equipment is not always available, drug users may have to share needles and equipment, which further contributes to the spread of infections. Significant resources are spent on law enforcement, money that could instead be spent on prevention and the expansion of treatment facilities for drug users.

The most pronounced effect, however, is that it pushes drug users to the margins of society. This makes it difficult to reach them with educational messages, makes users afraid to go to health or social services, may make service providers shy away from providing essential education on safer use

of drugs for fear of being seen as condoning use, and fosters antidrug attitudes toward the user, directing action toward punishment of the "offender"
rather than fostering understanding and assistance.

Programming to Deal with Drug and Alcohol Addiction

The Canadian Center on Substance Abuse estimates that substance abuse
cost more than $18.45 billion (U.S.$12 billion) in Canada in 1992. This
represents $649 (U.S.$422) per capita, or about 2.67 percent of the total
gross domestic product (Single et al. 1996, p. 6).

Alcohol accounts for more than $7.5 billion (U.S.$4.9 billion) in costs,
or $265 per capita. This represents 40.8 percent of the total costs of sub-
stance abuse. The largest economic costs of alcohol are $4.1 billion
(U.S.$2.7 billion) for lost productivity owing to illness and premature death,
$1.36 billion (U.S.$88 million) for law enforcement, and $1.3 billion
(U.S.$85 million) in direct health care costs. Tobacco accounts for $9.56
billion (U.S.$6.21 billion) in costs, or $336 (U.S.$218) per capita. This is
more than half (51.8 percent) of the total substance abuse costs. Lost productivity caused by illness and premature death accounts for more than $6.8
billion (U.S.$4.4 billion) of these costs, and direct health care costs owing
to smoking account for $2.67 billion (U.S.$1.74 billion). The economic
costs of illicit drugs are estimated at $1.37 billion (U.S.$90 million), or $48
(U.S.$17) per capita. The largest cost (approximately $823 million
[U.S.$535 million]) is lost productivity due to illness and premature death,
and substantial portions of the costs ($400 million [U.S.$144 million]) are
for law enforcement. Direct health care costs due to illicit drugs are estimated at $88 million (U.S.$52 million) (Single et al., 1996, p. 6).

HISTORY OF ALCOHOL AND DRUG USE IN CANADA

The legal framework of the current system of drug control in Canada was
laid down in the early part of the twentieth century. By 1908 all medicines,
as well as tobacco and alcohol, were on the way to regulation. In the same
year, the Opium Act created the first drug prohibition. Other opiates and
cocaine were covered in the Opium and Drug Act of 1911, and cannabis
was added in 1923. Antialcohol groups gained support during the first two
decades of the century, and all provinces enacted some form of alcohol
prohibition during World War I.

By 1929 all provinces except Prince Edward Island had rescinded alcohol
prohibition and imposed regulation of the alcohol trade. The Opium and
Narcotic Drug Act of 1929 was Canada's main instrument of drug policy
for the next forty years. International drug prohibition and regulation
through the Single Convention on Narcotic Drugs (1961) and the Con-

vention on Psychotropic Substances (1971), to which Canada was a signatory, have further reinforced the artificial division between legal and illegal—licit and illicit—drugs (Riley, 1998).

SUBSTANCE ABUSE IN CANADA TODAY

Political Views and Public Policies

More than one quarter of Canadians (27 percent) feel that the possession of small amounts of cannabis should be legal; 42 percent feel that possession should be against the law, but subject to either no penalty or a fine only for a first offense; and only 17 percent favor the current policy whereby a first offender is subject to a potential jail sentence. The remaining 14 percent have no opinion. Support for a more liberal cannabis policy is strongest among males, younger Canadians, and British Columbians (Single et al., 1998, p. 12).

According to the Canadian Center on Substance Abuse, Canada's drug strategy reflects a balance between reducing the supply of drugs and reducing the demand for drugs.

The strategy involves federal, provincial, and territorial governments and addiction agencies, nongovernmental organizations, professional associations, law enforcement agencies, the private sector, and community groups. The effectiveness of individual interventions is linked to the degree to which four principles have been recognized in development and implementation: sensitivity to gender, culture, and age; involvement of target groups; attention to the needs of drug users; and the underlying determinants associated with substance abuse.

In the future, the government intends to strengthen its prevention work responding to the needs of youth and young adults, enhance border interdiction activities, increase efforts to target the proceeds of crime and the property used to commit crimes, identify and assess innovative approaches to treatment and rehabilitation, and respond to the considerable harm associated with injection drug use.

At least two judicial decisions in Ontario and British Columbia have concluded that cannabis appears to be a much less dangerous drug for its consumers than either alcohol or tobacco. Deaths from alcohol and tobacco outstrip those from marijuana by a ratio of 10 to 1, even when relative rates of use are taken into account. Recent statistics (July 1998) show that, in 1997, there were 65,000 drug charges in Canada; 70 percent of these were related to cannabis use. More than 60 percent of all drug charges involve possession rather than distribution offenses. Therefore, the war against drugs in Canada remains primarily one against cannabis. "It is not surprising that there is a reluctance to give up this fight, as hypocritical and as futile as it must appear. Both sides in the war—the police and the marijuana distrib-utors—have nothing to gain and everything to lose if cannabis is given le-gitimacy as [a] recreational drug" (Riley, 1998, p. 26).

The most substantial legal change in relation to cannabis law occurred with the introduction of the Controlled Drugs and Substances Act. This legislation, for the first time, set marijuana apart from other illegal drugs. No longer a "narcotic," cannabis is now a Schedule II drug (cocaine and heroin are in Schedule I). The punishments for marijuana possession, dis-tribution, and production are slightly different from those for cocaine and heroin. If the amount of cannabis possessed is less than thirty grams (1.1 ounces) and the amount distributed is less than three kilograms (6.6 pounds), maximum jail terms are reduced to six months and five years, re-spectively. For heroin and cocaine, the maximum term for possession remains seven years, and the maximum term for distribution is life impris-onment.

These legal changes still support terms that are totally at odds with the norms seen in courts. While no dramatic changes in cannabis policy have occurred through legislation, changes have taken place through policing and the courts. By 1975 fines and discharges had emerged in Canadian courts as the most probable sanctions for marijuana possession. Data are no longer available regarding the rate of imprisonment for cannabis possession; fines and discharges remain the most common judicial response, both of which still incur a criminal record. More than 600,000 Canadians now have crim-inal records for marijuana possession. A number of attempts have been made to reduce the consequences of a drug offense, including pardons and dis-charges. The discharge provisions of the Criminal Code and the pardoning provisions of the Criminal Records Act in fact make little difference. A dis-charged offender might not be convicted but would have to admit that he or she had committed a criminal offense if questioned (such as when making border crossings) (Riley, 1998).

Harm Reduction

Harm reduction has emerged as an alternative approach to abstinence-oriented drug policy and programming. A significant degree of confusion and controversy has attended its rise to prominence. Harm reduction focuses on reducing the adverse consequences among persons who cannot be ex-pected to cease their use of drugs at the present time, but it can be com-patible with an eventual goal of abstention. This section attempts to clarify the issues regarding the definition and practice of harm reduction and makes recommendations to guide policy and program development.

Harm reduction, a public-health approach to dealing with drug-related issues, places priority on reducing the negative consequences of drug use rather than on eliminating drug use or ensuring abstinence. A primary catalyst for this surge of interest in harm reduction has been the emergence of AIDS, which is linked to drug use through the sharing of injection equipment. Many countries now take the public health–based perspective that the dangers of the spread of AIDS among drug users and from drug users into the general population pose a greater threat to health than the dangers of drug use itself.

At present, there is no agreement in the addiction literature or among practitioners as to the definition of harm reduction. Some harm-reduction advocates consider the reform of laws prohibiting drug possession to be an integral part of harm reduction; others do not. Some persons consider the imprisonment of drug users for simple possession to be a form of harm reduction. Practitioners dedicated to abstinence may also think of themselves as reducing the harms of substance abuse.

As these examples illustrate, there is considerable confusion and a lack of conceptual clarity concerning the meaning of harm reduction. It may help to clarify the term to distinguish between harm reduction as a goal and harm reduction as a strategy. As a general goal, virtually all drug policies and programs—including criminalization of users and abstinence-oriented programs—have a goal of harm reduction.

As a specific strategy, the term harm reduction generally refers only to those policies and programs that aim at reducing drug-related harm without requiring abstention from drug use. Using this definition, harm-reduction strategies would not include such strategies as abstinence-oriented treatment programs or the criminalization of illicit drug use. In other words, all drug policies and programs aim at reducing drug-related harm, but not all policies and programs with a goal of harm reduction are harm-reduction strategies.

Harm-reduction approaches are restricted to those strategies that place priority on reducing the negative consequences of drug use for the individual, the community, and society while the user continues to use drugs, at least for the present time. Harm-reduction approaches accept the use of drugs as a fact, and the focus is placed on reducing harm while use continues. A harm-reduction approach in the short term does not rule out abstinence in the long term. Indeed, harm-reduction approaches are often the first step toward the eventual cessation of drug use.

The essence of harm reduction is embodied in the following statement: If a person is not willing to give up his or her drug use, we should assist him or her in reducing harm to himself or herself and others.

The main characteristics or principles of harm reduction are pragmatism, humanistic values, focus on harms, and priority of immediate goals.

Pragmatism

Harm reduction accepts that some use of mind-altering substances is a common feature of human experience. It acknowledges that, while carrying risks, drug use also provides the user with benefits that must be taken into account if drug-using behavior is to be understood. From a community perspective, containment and amelioration of drug-related harms may be a more pragmatic or feasible option than efforts to eliminate drug use entirely.

Humanistic Values

The drug user's decision to use drugs is accepted as fact. This does not mean that drug use is condoned. No moralistic judgment is made either to condemn or to support use of drugs, regardless of the level of use or the mode of intake. The dignity and rights of the drug user are respected.

Focus on Harms

The fact or extent of a person's drug use per se is of secondary importance to the risk of harms consequent to use. The harms addressed can be related to health, social, economic, or a multitude of other factors, which affect the individual, the community, and society as a whole. Therefore, the first priority is to decrease the negative consequences of drug use to the user and to others, as opposed to focusing on decreasing the drug use itself. Harm reduction neither excludes nor presumes the long-term treatment goal of abstinence. In some cases, reduction of level of use may be one of the most effective forms of harm reduction. In others, alteration in the mode of use (i.e., from injecting to smoking) may be more effective.

Priority of Immediate Goals

Most harm-reduction programs have a hierarchy of goals, with the immediate focus on proactively engaging individuals, target groups, and communities to address their most pressing needs. Achieving immediate and realistic goals is usually viewed as the first step toward risk-free use, or, if appropriate, abstinence.

Examples of Harm-Reduction Programs and Policies
Syringe Exchange and Availability

Many people regard needle- and syringe-exchange programs as the epitome of the harm-reduction approach. These programs were first established in the Netherlands in the mid-1980s. By the end of the decade, clinics were operating in numerous cities around the world. The rationale behind syringe exchanges is that many people who are currently injecting are unable or unwilling to stop, and intervention strategies must help reduce their risk of HIV infection and transmission to others. Provision of sterile needles and syringes is a simple, inexpensive way to reduce the risk of spreading the HIV infection. It is also a way of providing contact with drug users through outreach services.

In Amsterdam, police stations provide clean syringes on an exchange basis. Automated syringe-exchange machines are now being used in many European and Australian cities. These vending machines release a clean syringe when a used one is deposited. Such machines are fairly inexpensive and accessible on a twenty-four hour basis. The machines, however, decrease the important personal contact between drug users and health-care workers.

Bleach kits, which contain bleach and instructions for cleaning equipment, can be distributed as another way to make drug injection less dangerous. Although bleach is not totally effective in eliminating HIV and it does not kill the pathogen that causes hepatitis, such kits do help reduce the likelihood of an infection's being passed by the sharing of dirty equipment.

In Canada, there are now more than 100 syringe exchanges, with more being established at the present time. In a number of provinces, pharmacists are becoming actively involved in syringe-exchange programs. There is now clear evidence that attendance at syringe exchanges and increased syringe availability is associated with a decrease in risk (e.g., decreased sharing) as well as a decrease in harm (e.g., lower levels of HIV infection).

Methadone Programs

Numerous studies have shown that methadone maintenance reduces morbidity and mortality, diminishes the users' involvement in crime, curbs the spread of HIV, and helps drug users gain control of their lives. One of the key factors underlying the success of methadone as a harm-reduction measure is that it brings the user back into the community rather than treating him or her like an outsider or a criminal. Methadone programs work best if they are numerous, accessible, and flexible. Further expansion of methadone programs should take into account the need for such programs in prisons as well as the advantages of offering methadone treatment as an alternative to imprisonment and other forms of criminalization.

Education and Outreach Programs

Drug education materials with a harm-reduction focus aimed at high-risk populations are readily available. However, such educational materials remain extremely controversial. Although they do not promote drug use, such materials tell the user how to reduce the risks associated with using drugs, teaching such things as safer injecting practices. In some countries, such as the United Kingdom, these techniques are taught by nurses at clinics.

In many countries, outreach workers contact persons such as drug injectors and prostitutes at risk of becoming infected with HIV. These workers distribute educational material, syringes, condoms, and bleach kits and help users contact other services.

Law Enforcement Policies

One of the most important features of police strategy has been to place priority on the enforcement of laws against drug trafficking while using a "cautioning" policy toward drug use. Cautioning involves taking an offender to a police station, confiscating the drug, recording the incident, and formally warning the offender that any further unlawful possession of drugs will result in prosecution in court. The offender must also meet certain conditions, such as not having a previous drug conviction and not having an extensive criminal record. The person is also given information about treatment services in the area, including syringe exchanges. The first time an offender is cautioned, he or she is not given a criminal record. On the second and third occasions, offenders are sent to court. If an addict becomes registered through a service agency, then he or she is legally entitled to carry drugs for personal use. The overall effect of this policy is to steer users away from crime and possible imprisonment. Cautioning has been recommended by the United Kingdom's attorney general as an appropriate option for cannabis possession.

In Canada, the general approach toward drug use has been criminalization, although diversion of users to treatment is increasingly employed. The recent shift toward community policing in a number of cities may permit the application of more harm-reduction measures by local enforcement authorities in the near future.

Tolerance Areas

Several European cities have developed facilities known as "tolerance zones," "injection rooms," "health rooms," or "contact centers," where drug users can get together and obtain clean injection equipment, condoms, advice, and medical attention. These tolerance areas are often motivated by harm reduction, but they may serve other purposes, such as social control and urban beautification. Most of these places allow users to remain anonymous. Some include space where drug users, including injectors, can take drugs in a comparatively safe environment. This is regarded as better than the open injection of illicit drugs in public places or consumption of drugs in "shooting galleries," which are usually unhygienic and controlled by drug dealers.

Alcohol Policies and Programs

Harm reduction has been a common approach to the prevention and treatment of alcohol problems. Prevention programs, such as the designated driver programs aimed at preventing impaired driving, are harm-reduction measures in that they aim to reduce the harms associated with alcohol use without necessarily requiring abstention. With regard to treatment, controlled drinking programs attempt to teach people to consume alcohol in a moderate or sensible manner. A number of programs have been designed for problem drinkers.

THE FUTURE OF SUBSTANCE ABUSE IN CANADA

Much of the cost of illicit drugs in Canada is attributable to policing and the criminal justice system. Yet studies have repeatedly shown that prevention and treatment are far more cost-effective than are approaches that depend on criminal law. Methadone and other forms of treatment can cut down on the amount spent on illegal drugs and can reduce the crimes committed to obtain drugs. Treatment can also reduce other criminal behavior through reducing alcohol and drug use. The result is a saving not only in terms of economic loss due to theft but also in terms of legal and prison costs. Drug treatment is a more cost-effective method than confinement for reducing drug use and crime: about two-thirds of the benefit for one-tenth of the annual cost (Riley, 1998, p. 56). Such reduction in criminal behavior, however, occurs only as long as the user stays in treatment and only as long as the treatment is effective. The effectiveness of the treatment and whether the user stays in treatment depend on the type of treatment offered. Flexible treatment programs, where multiple options exist for each person, appear to be the most effective in keeping users away from illegal drugs and the most successful at retaining clients (Riley, 1998).

Alternatives to the current approach to drug use and drug users in Canada are possible. Alternatives within the current prohibitionist policy that would not require any changes to the current legal framework could include the de facto decriminalization of cannabis possession for personal use, medical prescription of heroin, explicit educational programs, and so on. Alternatives to the current prohibitionist approach may require that Canada denounce several international drug-control conventions.

CONCLUSION

The problems that are related to criminalizing drug users have not been addressed. Criminalization increases the social and economic costs and fails to reduce drug availability. The criminal approach to drug use increases rather than decreases harm from drug use. Harm reduction has emerged as an alternative approach to abstinence-oriented drug policy and programming. Much of the cost of illicit drugs in Canada is attributable to policing and the criminal justice system. Treatment can reduce criminal behavior through reducing alcohol and drug use as well as the costs associated with the criminal justice system. Alternatives to the current approach to drug use and drug users in Canada are possible.

REFERENCES

Conley, P., Hewitt, D., Mitic, W., Poulin, C., Riley, D., Room, R., Sawka, E., Single, E., and Topp, J. (1993). *"Harm reduction: Concepts and practice, a policy discussion paper.*" Paper presented at the Fifth International Conference on the Reduction of Drug-Related Harm. Toronto.

Jackson, Greg. (1996, June 26). Statistics silent on pain of addiction. *The Press* (Canterbury, New Zealand), p. 22.

Reed, Maureen, and Hiebert, Daniel. Canada. *Microsoft Encarta Encyclopedia*, 2000 edition.

Riley, Diane. (1998). *Drug and drug policy in Canada: A brief review and commentary.* Ottawa: Canadian Foundation for Drug Policy.

Single, E., Fischer, B., Room, R., Poulin, C., Sawka, E., Thompson, H., and Topp, J. (1998, May). "Cannabis control in Canada: Options regarding possession." A Canadian Center on Substance Abuse policy discussion document prepared by the CCSA national working group on addictions policy.

Single, E., Robson, L., Xie, X., and Rehm, J. (1996). *The Costs of Substance Abuse in Canada.* Canadian Center on Substance Abuse, 75 Albert Street, Suite 300, Ottawa, Ontario, Canada K1P 5E7.

Smart, R.G. (1983). *Forbidden highs: The nature, treatment, and prevention of illicit drug abuse.* Toronto: Addiction Research Foundation.

Statistics Canada (1996–97). *National Population Health Survey.* Toronto: Federal Publications, Inc.

3

CHINA

Andrew Cherry

INTRODUCTION

The drug problem in China helps drive drug production, trafficking, addiction, and the spread of HIV/AIDS in Southeast Asia. At a distance, the heroin trade in Southeast Asia has no borders, but the heroin trade region is clearly an identifiable region of Southeast Asia. Not just one or two Asian countries are involved in the heroin trade, which many would suggest. Instead, the drug trade flourishes across borders with virtual impunity because of corrupt governments, politicians, armies, international corporations, and other legitimate-looking organizations that launder the money and move it from one bank to another, from one country to another, until it is impossible to trace its sources.

The illegal drug industry in Southeast Asia respects no borders, and it recognizes no laws but the law of supply and demand. When the sophistication of the Southeast Asian heroin industry business strategy is revealed, it is quite clear that the business strategies used by the British in marketing opium to the Chinese in the 1700s and 1800s have not been lost on modern-day Asian, illegal drug-cartel leaders.

Chinese officials deny corruption in the national government; however, at the local level, both drug trafficking and drug using are widespread along the border shared with Burma and Thailand. Drug use and drug trafficking can also lead to death if wrongdoers are caught by the wrong official.

China's history has numerous accounts of pandemic opium addiction. Probably no other country in the world has suffered more at the hands of addictive drugs—with the possible exception of Colombia and the more recent example of Russia with its people's crippling addiction to alcohol.

The British imported opium into China in the eighteenth and nineteenth centuries, despite the ban on opium trade that was imposed in China by the Chinese government in 1800. This ban was ignored by Britain, and the Chinese government was forced to allow the British to continue selling opium in China, making enormous profits into the late 1800s. The mass opium addiction among the Chinese in the eighteenth and nineteenth centuries destroyed the Chinese economy and its people, especially in the country's south (Tho'Mas, 1997). These facts may explain why the Chinese attitude toward illegal drug use and drug trafficking inside China is so harsh. It may also explain why, for years, the Chinese government only paid lip service to calls from the Western world to stop drugs from moving out of China or through China. Chinese officials may have felt it was tit for tat.

In midsummer 2000, a new antidrug campaign, based on a show-no-mercy policy to traffickers and users, was launched in China. In one week in July 2000 almost 50 drug traffickers and dealers were executed, shot in the back of the head, nationwide in China. A blaze of publicity accompanied the executions (Media Awareness Project, 2000).

Although Chinese civilization outpaced the rest of the world in the arts and sciences for centuries, in the first half of the twentieth century, China was beset by major famines, civil unrest, military defeats, and foreign occupation. After World War II, the Communists under Mao Zedong gained control of the mainland after the National Chinese Army fled to the island of Formosa. While Communist party control ensured China's sovereignty, it also imposed strict controls over everyday life and particularly the use of opium. Opium use was prohibited in 1946, and the prohibition was enforced with severe punishment for opium users. Death was a common consequence for selling and continuing to use opium after several warnings. The abuse of narcotics was eventually eliminated for the most part; however, there was an accommodation for the elderly. Those elderly who had been smoking opium most of their lives were allowed to continue to smoke opium, but no new users were allowed to go unpunished if caught. Because of the threat, many addicts in the south of China migrated to Hong Kong, which increased the opium addict population there for some years (Central Intelligence Agency, 2000a).

Fifty years after Communist China declared the narcotic problem solved in China, the Chinese again faced a problem with illegal drugs. Although denial of social problems was the norm among Chinese officials, there was exceptional frankness about the impact of the drug trade and drug abuse in the year 2000. In June 2000, the Chinese government issued a white paper, *Narcotics Control in China*, which outlines the extent of the problem within China. The white paper was the official declaration to begin again the task of controlling illegal drugs.

According to official Chinese documents, there are roughly 681,000 registered drug addicts in China, and most of them are addicted to heroin. In the 1980s, they were reporting about 150,000 addicts. The white paper was motivated by growing concern that if the Chinese government did not start cooperating with other nations to control the heroin problem in Southeast Asia, the drug problem could spread like an epidemic in China. Consequently, in 1999, the amount of illegal drugs seized by Chinese authorities rose by 33 percent. Over the year, 5.3 tons of heroin, 1.2 tons of opium, 16 tons of methamphetamines, and smaller amounts of cocaine and marijuana were seized and impounded by Chinese authorities. "It is highly necessary to strengthen international cooperation in drug control to promote the battle against narcotics worldwide and radically solve the drug problem in China," the paper states. To implement the white paper's propositions, the Chinese increased their cooperation with bordering countries and with the international community. In 2000 China signed drug intelligence cooperation agreements with the United States which provide for the sharing of information between Chinese police and the Federal Bureau of Investigation (FBI) (Media Awareness Project, 2000).

A Brief Profile of China

China is located in East Asia, south of Russia and Mongolia. One of the world's largest countries in land area, it is the largest country in terms of population. The capital city of Communist China is Beijing, and the largest city is Shanghai. China has more than 3,400 offshore islands. The total landmass is approximately 3,700,000 square miles (about 9,580,000 square kilometers). Although Communist China claims Taiwan, Taiwan has refused to recognize the authority of the Communist government of the People's Republic of China since 1949.

Mainland China's climate is extremely diverse. There are tropical conditions in the south and subarctic conditions in the north. The highest point in China is Mount Everest at 29,028 feet above sea level. Even though China has a great landmass, little of it is farmland. Only 10 percent of China's land can be farmed; 43 percent is in pastures, and another 14 percent is forest and woodland (*Encarta Desk Encyclopedia*, 1998).

Air pollution and acid rain (caused by greenhouse gases, sulfur dioxide particulates) are serious problems in China which are the result of China's heavy reliance on coal. There are also water shortages in the north of China. Water pollution from untreated sewage is a problem throughout China. Deforestation continues, and it has been estimated that 20 percent of China's agricultural land was lost between 1950 and 2000 to soil erosion and economic development. Trade in endangered species (such as tiger bones, cobra skins, and rhino parts) continues to be practiced in China with little government interference.

The population of China is over one and a quarter billion people (1,261,832,482, according to the July 2000 estimate). The birthrate is slightly over 16 births per 1,000 people. The death rate is less than 6.75 deaths per 1,000 people as estimated in 2000. The infant mortality rate was 28.92 deaths per 1,000 live births in the year 2000. The sex ratio, which is important because of the one child, one family policy in China, in 2000, was 1.15 boys for every girl born in China. There were 1.1 boys for every girl under fifteen years of age and 1.06 males for every female between fifteen and sixty-four years of age. At sixty-five years of age, the ratio switches. The ratio between men and women for those sixty-five and older is 0.88 males for every female. For the total population, however, the ratio is 1.06 males for every female in the year 2000. The life expectancy at birth in the year 2000 was 69.6 years for males and 73.33 years for females (Central Intelligence Agency, 2000b).

Almost 92 percent of the people living in China are ethnic Han Chinese. The remaining 8 percent of the population comprises Zhuang, Uygur, Hui, Yi, Tibetan, Miao, Manchu, Mongol, Buyi, Korean, and other nationalities. The Chinese people practice the religions of Daoism (Taoism), Buddhism, Islam (2%–3%), and Christianity (1%). The government officially recognizes only atheism (Central Intelligence Agency, 2000b).

As defined by the Communist Chinese government, 81.5 percent of the people who are fifteen years of age or older can read and write: 89.9 percent of males and 72.7 percent of females (a 1995 estimate). The GDP (purchasing power) was $4.8 trillion (U.S. dollars as estimated in 1999). The per capita GPA was $3,800 (estimated in 1999). Roughly 10 percent of the population lived below the poverty level. There were 700 million (a 1998 estimate) in China's labor force. About 50 percent of the people work in agriculture, 24 percent work in industry, and about 26 percent work in the service industry. The unemployment rate was steady at around 10 percent, but it was often higher in rural areas (as estimated in 1999) [Central Intelligence Agency, 2000b].

In general, China is a large country struggling with the problem of an ever-increasing population. Even though China's potential for serious problems is great, there is an equally good chance of China's having a prosperous future.

VIGNETTE

When police officers raided a rundown flat in the North Point area of Hong Kong in 1991, they discovered one of the few remaining opium dens in the world. The three occupants arrested were elderly male pensioners.

A search of the Java Road apartment turned up the traditional apparatus that had been used by Hong Kong's opium addicts since opium was introduced as the centerpiece of Britain's diplomacy and trade policy with China. The police confiscated worn, stained opium pipes and lamps. The police also found 44 grams of opium, and a small amount of opium water.

The owner of the flat, eighty-year-old Ho Yuen, pleaded guilty at Eastern Magistracy to three counts relating to the manufacture of opium and running a *divan*, the official term for where opium is sold or smoked. Ho Yuen was sentenced to jail for four weeks. The judge also fined his two customers who were arrested at the opium den: Lai Tak-hung, age seventy-two, $600 (U.S.) and Lam Chee-hing, eighty-three, $300 (U.S.). The duty lawyer reported that all three were pensioners who were living on $425 (U.S.) a month and had been opium addicts since the 1930s and 1940s.

When the last of these old-time opium addicts dies, opium addiction will also die out. Most of the remaining opium users, like the three arrested, are old men who have been addicted since World War II.

Why did opium die out as the primary drug of addiction after alcohol? It was not because people quit using narcotics. Drug addicts turned away from opium to heroin because heroin is more potent and easier to use than opium, and, for the producer and trafficker, the profits are far greater for the same risks (Dobson, 1992).

OVERVIEW OF SUBSTANCE ABUSE IN CHINA WITH BASIC DEMOGRAPHICS

Because China is closed to outsiders and because the government maintains a tight control on the media, there is little information about the extent of the substance-abuse problem in China. However, there is convincing evidence of substance abuse along its western borders. The Chinese province of Yunnan is located on the Chinese side of the border. The border with Burma is shared by the Kachin and Shan states. Yunnan Province, in 2000, had the highest prevalence rate of HIV infection in the People's Republic of China. The Chinese Ministry of Health reported that 80.4 percent (1,426 of a total of 1,774) of all HIV infections in China were in Yunnan, and 60 percent of all confirmed AIDS cases were in Yunnan Province (Wu, Detels, and Zhang, 1995). Additionally, the HIV infection rate in 1994 in the Chinese border district of Ruili, across from the Kachin State of Burma, was 62 percent among drug users who injected. The majority of these drug users were ethnic Kachin (Jingpo in Chinese) and Wa. Chinese authorities were more open about illegal drugs crossing over from Burma and Thailand than about drugs or HIV/AIDS problems in the heart of China. Even so, Chinese officials, who may have blamed Burma for their heroin problem, did not explicitly link heroin trafficking to the Burma military junta because Burma was an ally in world politics (Chinese Ministry of Health and UNAIDS Programme, 1997).

HISTORY OF ALCOHOL AND DRUG USE IN CHINA

In the entire world, no country has suffered more at the hands of addictive drugs than China. Yet, these drug problems did not exist in China before European colonials used it to destroy China's culture and economy. Traditional use of opium had never been a problem in China. Opium was first used in Chinese medicine in the late 1400s. The Chinese used opium effectively to treat dysentery, cholera, and other diseases. There were no reports of opium problems among the Chinese until the 1700s. Nonetheless, when it did appear, it spread quickly. By 1729 Chinese imperial officials were so alarmed at the growing numbers of opium users and the debilitating effect of opium on the users, that they prohibited the sale of opium-laced tobacco and banned opium dens. Selling opium for smoking was considered a crime in the same class as robbery and murder, and it was punishable by banishment or death.

The threat of such harsh punishment, however, did not stop the British opium tradesmen. In the late 1700s, the British started gradually to take over the Chinese opium trade from Portugal and Holland. This was possible because most of the opium sold in China at the time was grown in India, which was under the control of the British. In the late 1700s, the Indian city of Patna was the home to both English and Dutch opium-processing plants. There were reports that the large opium-processing plants in Patna produced enough opium to meet the needs for all of India. The opium produced in other areas of India provided great profits for the British East India Company.

Britain's Opium Trade

While the Chinese government was taking stronger measures to end the opium trade and abuse, the British were doing all they could to increase the opium trade in China. To this end, Britain's East India Company waged three wars against the Chinese government to secure the right to sell opium in China. The first Opium War was the world's first drug war. The sole purpose of the opium war was to secure a market in China so that the East India Company could continue to sell a corrosive, addictive substance (opium) in China. The opium trade was extremely lucrative for the British, but it destroyed the lives of millions of Chinese citizens.

Opium sales rose gradually in China from 2,330 chests in 1788 to 4,968 chests in 1810. Once the British had the monopoly, however, they pushed sales up to 17,257 chests by 1835. There was so much confidence in the stability of the opium trade in China that, in 1830, the British governor-general of India wrote, "We are taking measures for extending the cultivation of the poppy, with a view to a large increase in the supply of opium" (Tho'Mas, 1997).

The first Opium War started in 1839 when Chinese imperial government troops confronted foreign merchant ships and demanded the British surrender their illegal cargo of opium. The imperial officials then ordered thousands of confiscated chests of opium burned. When the superintendent of the British fleet heard of the destruction of British property, he ordered the governor-general of India to send as many ships as could be spared to China to defend British solvency. The ships were sent to Hong Kong, where they protected the opium-carrying British merchant vessels in and out of that major southern Chinese port. The emperor sent Chinese junks to drive off the British fleet, but they were no match for the British warships. The wars waged against China caused untold deaths and casualties. The British destroyed, plundered, looted, and raped cities and towns along the coast of China. By this time, the few remnants of compassion for humankind had been swept away like the Chinese junks to allow the continued unrestricted flow of enormous profits from the sale of opium.

The *India Gazette*, a British publication, wrote about the sack of Chusan in 1840, during the first Opium War. The article reported that every house was broken into and looted, and that the looting did not stop until there was nothing left to take or destroy. The first Opium War ended on August 29, 1842, and the Treaty of Nanking forced the Chinese government to pay $15 million to the British merchants, open up five Chinese ports to unrestricted English trade, and surrender Hong Kong to the British. This was the origin of British rule in Hong Kong.

Following the Opium War

After the first Opium War, Chinese officials continued to look for ways to end the British opium trade in China. They were diplomatically and militarily too weak to stop British opium traffickers. At the same time, the British continued to ship increasing amounts of Indian opium into China.

As China's government continued to resist the British opium trade, it went more into debt to Britain. In addition to the money it owed the British for having lost the first Opium War, China was later required to pay the costs of foreign troops who were needed to end the Taiping Rebellion which broke out in 1850. While putting down the rebellion, foreign troops damaged large areas of China, and as many as 30 million people may have died in the fighting. China's continued opposition to the British opium trade only resulted in Britain's intensifying its demand that China's interior be opened to Western trade.

A second Opium War broke out in 1856, and again China lost the war. In 1858 the Chinese signed another trade agreement that placed a small tax on imported opium. This agreement began a forty-eight-year period of a de facto legalization of the domestic cultivation of opium, as well as the importation of opium.

This agreement resulted in the domestic cultivation of opium, and the cultivation of opium spread quickly in China. At first, in the 1860s, domestic or homegrown opium was considered inferior to Indian opium. Nonetheless, it was cheaper and its quality rapidly improved. In many areas, it sold for less than half the price of the foreign smoking opium. Moreover, the poppy was a valuable crop for Chinese peasants. Raw opium sold for two to four times what one could get for wheat. The low weight and bulk of opium made it easier to transport over rough terrain, tempting to small farmers in areas where trade routes were often narrow, winding trails.

In the peak year of 1880 China imported more than 6,500 tons of opium, most of which was produced in India. However, after 1880, the demand for foreign opium decreased, and by 1905, the amount of opium imported was roughly 3,250 tons. At the same time, China's annual opium crop was over 22,000 tons (DrugTexT Foundation, 1996; Inglis, 1975).

History of the Development of the Golden Triangle

In the mid-1800s the mountainous provinces of Szechwan and Yunnan (part of the Golden Triangle) were located where the farmers found advantageous to grow a lightweight crop worth more than traditional grains on the open market. These provinces, a thousand miles from a weakened central government in Peking, were well suited for poppy cultivation. Yunnan Province, which borders Burma, Laos, and Tonkin (now part of northern Vietnam), became an opium producer second only to the western province of Szechwan. While the central government received relatively little from taxes on the cultivation and sale of domestic opium, revenue from the drug trade became a mainstay of the provincial economy. In 1875 over 33 percent of the farmable land of Yunnan Province was planted in opium poppy. Opium was Yunnan's most important product in total exports by 1903, and it continued to be one of Yunnan's most lucrative exports in 2000 (DrugTexT Foundation, 1996; Inglis, 1975; Holley, 1990).

Before the Europeans colonized Southeast Asia, there were few rigid borders in what has become known as the Golden Triangle. From Burma to the Tonkin region, the China–Southeast Asia frontier was sparsely populated by diverse ethnic groups distinct both from the ethnic Han Chinese and from the dominant Southeast Asian ethnic groups. It is impossible to know when the isolated tribal groups along this frontier first began to cultivate opium poppies. However, as an opium-poppy cultivation area, the Golden Triangle went largely unnoticed as a producer of opium until the late 1800s; at that time, its production of opium was dwarfed by Chinese and British Indian production. After World War II, the Golden Triangle became a player in the international narcotic drug-trafficking business. During the Vietnam War, it flourished as an opium-producing area.

British Business Interest Conflicts with National Morality

Toward the end of the 1800s, the moral outrage expressed by many of Britain's intellectuals and missionaries from around the world was having an effect on the British government. To deal with the condemnation, the British government established the British Royal Commission on Opium. In 1894 the commission concluded with a report that declared that prohibiting the cultivation of opium would place a considerable financial burden on the Indian taxpayer, who would have to compensate the government for the loss of the opium revenue. Furthermore, they concluded, it would not help for Britain to stop opium production as long as China's government was too weak to suppress the demand for opium. Accusations against the traffickers by those familiar with the Chinese situation were largely ignored. The question, as the commission saw it, was not how to eliminate Indian production but whether to do so, and the answer, as usual, was no. Opium was too profitable to be abandoned (Inglis, 1975; Holley, 1990). These conclusions, which did not satisfy the antiopium movement, did not alter the fact that Chinese production of opium was making Britain's opium trade less and less profitable.

In 1900, after a hundred years of British opium trade, there were 15 million Chinese opium addicts. Many of the Chinese addicts used opium to forget or ignore the painful realities of their hopeless lives. The craving to continue smoking, regardless of the cost, added yet another element to the misery. Although some of the very rich could afford both opium and food, many family fortunes literally went up in smoke, and the impoverished addicts often died of starvation. The Chinese government could not stop opium addiction even in their own ranks. Candidates for office in the Chinese government were reported to have died from the effects of withdrawal during the arduous three-day examinations. A Western observer on a trip to Szechwan complained that all but two of her 143 official escorts were "on the pipe." Twice she reported being forced to wait to have her passport registered because the scribes were recovering from their "narcotic siesta." Despite the extensive sorrow and suffering caused by opium, everyone knew that opium was the ultimate cure for the realities that overwhelmed even the strongest; swallowing an overdose of opium was a popular method of committing suicide (Inglis, 1975; Holley, 1990).

As opium addiction spread throughout Asia, across Europe, and into the United States, organized opposition to Britain's part in the Chinese opium trade grew stronger and more verbal. Missionaries complained that addiction among the "heathen" Chinese made the task of converting them to Christianity much more difficult. The Chinese regarded missionaries and foreign drug traffickers as intruders selling goods that disrupted their society and violated their culture. Thus, missionaries and opium were often linked in the minds of Chinese as different aspects of a single, "foreign menace" (DrugTexT Foundation, 1996).

China's political star continued to fall into the twentieth century. A humiliating defeat by Japan in the war of 1894–1895 led to internal demands for sweeping changes in the government. Western retaliation against the Chinese government for the destruction caused by the Boxer Rebellion in 1899–1900 exacerbated the deterioration of the country. China's military had been badly beaten time after time, and the government was forced to accept increasing burdensome financial obligations to pay for reparation.

The last Opium War convinced the imperial court and China's intellectuals that China must accept the opium trade if China were to survive. Opium was a clear-cut symptom and a glaring symbol of foreign intrusion and national decay. The opium trade, however, persisted in China. The endurance of the opium trade can be illustrated by a report published in 1951 by the United Nations. The United Nations Economic and Social Council issued a proclamation calling for Communist China to stop its attempt to sell a shipment of 500 tons of opium which was sitting on a Hong Kong dock (United Nations, Economic and Social Council, 1951).

SUBSTANCE ABUSE IN CHINA TODAY

In the early 1980s heroin abuse, which had been spreading for years, seemed to be leveling off in response to concerted national and international efforts. However, by the 1990s, heroin addiction was again on the rise and spreading across Southeast Asia and into neighboring countries from Burma and Thailand, including China and India.

Political Views and Public Policies

The attraction of narcotics and alcohol cannot be fully understood; however, certain public policies tend to increase its use and abuse. For instance, prohibition policies heighten the awareness and attraction of illegal drugs. Under prohibition, drug use tends to increase. Yet, while prohibition policies have failed in the rest of the world, they succeeded in Communist China, at least the last half of the twentieth century, when illegal drug use virtually soared in the rest of the world. Although it was losing its iron grip on its citizens' lives in 2000, especially along its western borders, China's prohibition policy against opium and heroin was the one case in which the prohibition of drugs succeeded, if only for a short time. The question is how did the Communists stamp out the drug problem in China? Before the Communists took control of China, colonialism and opium had almost destroyed the country. By the mid-1950s there were few reports of opium being used at all in China outside of its role in traditional medicine.

The problem with this archetype of prohibition, however, is the question: Was the cure worse than the ailment?

Three major forces facilitated Mao Zedong's prohibition against opium and heroin. The first factor was public opinion. In China, public opinion was against opium. It was viewed as a part of a larger foreign conspiracy to destroy China and its people. Second, China's society was so communalized that no one had any privacy. It was nearly impossible for those who smoked opium to smoke for any length of time without being caught and denounced by a neighbor or family member. It was even harder for Chinese farmers to cultivate poppies. Third, and paramount, was the fact that opium smuggling into China was stopped. The Chinese officials took the profit out of opium smuggling by shutting down ordinary commercial channels through which opium could be illicitly distributed (Inglis, 1975).

Much like the Chinese, people in most countries view illegal drugs as a threat to their society. Nevertheless, the concern and fear of illegal drugs is offset by the desire for individual privacy and freedom of movement. Illegal drugs in some quantity can be smuggled into most countries because of the freedom of movement between countries. Individual privacy also allows illegal drug transactions to occur without scrutiny. Individual privacy also allows those who are able to obtain illegal drugs to take them with relatively little exposure or risk (Inglis, 1975). China's model of prohibition will not work in countries with less draconian control. Consequently, as long as most countries permit their citizens to retain economic and social freedoms, the Chinese model for prohibiting substance abuse will not succeed.

Social Views, Customs, and Practices

Because China shares its border with countries that make up the Golden Triangle, opium has become a cross-border problem. Since the 1970s and the Vietnam War, a major proportion of the opium produced in the Golden Triangle areas of Burma, Laos, and Thailand have passed through Chinese provinces and cities in the northeast of China. The opium is transported to Eastern European markets and then distributed to Western Europe and the United States. This trade has resulted in a boom to the local economies of these Chinese provinces, but it has also resulted in a swelling number of heroin addicts and new HIV/AIDS cases (Associated Press, 1997). Because some of the opium and heroin is used to pay for services from Chinese traffickers and because these drugs are sold in local markets, the heroin trade that started in the 1970s has resulted in a growing drug problem in China in 2000.

The People's War on Drugs in China

In the late 1980s and 1990s, given some loosening up of economic control by the central government, China experienced an economic boom.

Likewise, it also brought with it an increase in drug use and abuse. Estimates in the late 1990s suggest that nearly 500,000 Chinese under the age of thirty-five were addicted to hard drugs, such as heroin and methamphetamines (Ozanich, 1997). In response to this new wave of addiction, in 1997, Chinese officials launched what was called a "people's war against drugs." The drug crackdown in the 1990s in China was similar to its antidrug campaign in the 1950s. For those who were addicted, there was mandatory drug treatment. For drug dealers and traffickers, the punishment was execution. In the 1950s, in the early years of the Communist era, those policies all but eliminated drug use in China. Yet, China is a vastly different country than it was in the 1950s. Nevertheless, Chinese officials say they are determined to stop a repeat of the widespread opium addiction that battered Chinese society prior to the Communists coming to power in 1949. "Today, in our socialist country under the leadership of the Chinese Communist Party, we would never allow drugs to spread unchecked," said a spokesperson of the Beijing Anti-Drug Committee (Ozanich, 1997). Lending its full support to China's war on drugs, the state-run television network routinely broadcasts footage of police drug crackdowns and executions of drug dealers. At the end of the twentieth century, heroin was still China's biggest drug problem, due largely to its proximity to the Golden Triangle. However, methamphetamines and Ecstasy were becoming more popular, particularly among young people in China's cities where the economy was booming and the influence of the West was potent among the young.

Drug Treatment in China

Compulsory drug treatment programs in China combine discipline and indoctrination about the harmfulness of drugs. At the Beijing Compulsory Drug Rehabilitation Center, patients are subjected to a regimen that combines the medical care of a hospital with the discipline of a prison. Patients are dressed identically in blue-and-white striped uniforms. Rehabilitation lasts from three to six months, during which time exercise and close monitoring of patients are a part of the daily routine.

The first two weeks are typically the toughest for most patients. It takes about two weeks to get over the sickness and physical discomfort associated with withdrawal from a physical dependency on heroin. Treatment requires patients to sit through countless lectures on drug laws while they are being swamped with antidrug propaganda. On the wall in front of them hangs, written in red letters, the slogan, "Forced drug abstention in accordance with the law." Additionally, compulsory drug treatment in China is very expensive. It costs most patients or their families more than half a year's salary (Ozanich, 1997).

THE FUTURE OF SUBSTANCE ABUSE IN CHINA

The next phase of China's drug history will be related to the experiences of Hong Kong and Taiwan, as they merge with the mainland Chinese government. How the reintegration of Hong Kong is handled will do a great deal to either speed up or slow down any reunion of Taiwan with China. The drug problem in Hong Kong and Taiwan is a significant one, and it has been handled much differently in these two regions than in mainland China.

Hong Kong

As one of Asia's dominant financial centers, even under Communist China's rule, Hong Kong continues to play a major role in providing international drug cartels access to laundered drug money needed to operate drug enterprises. Similarly, Hong Kong's geographical location, in proximity to the Golden Triangle and southern China, has always made this area an ideal location for the illegal transshipment of narcotics. Between January and October 1998, 8,150 individuals were arrested for drug-related offenses in Hong Kong. This number of arrests suggests that there is a serious drug problem in Hong Kong. When the number arrested is added to the amount of drugs confiscated, it makes a convincing argument that a sizable drug problem exists. Between January and November 1998, Hong Kong narcotics officers seized 176.65 kilograms (389.4 lbs.) of heroin, 2.17 kilograms (4.78 lbs.) of opium, 12.72 kilograms (28 lbs.) of cocaine, 521 kilograms (1,149 lbs.) of cannabis (herbal), 44.4 kilograms (97.9 lbs.) of cannabis (resin), and 231 kilograms (509 lbs.) of methamphetamines (Central Intelligence Agency, 2000a).

Given these circumstances, Hong Kong in 1998 had an active prevention and education program designed to discourage drug use, particularly among the young. The primary aim was to heighten the public's awareness of the undesirable consequences of abusing drugs, whether labeled "hard" or "soft." In 1998 about $45 million (U.S.) was spent on prevention programming (Dobson, 1992; Central Intelligence Agency, 2000a).

Taiwan

Taiwan is not involved in the cultivation or production of illegal narcotics, but the people of Taiwan use both heroin and methamphetamines, a problem which continued into the year 2000. Taiwan is also a transit point for drugs which eventually wind up in the United States. It has had an important role as a regional transportation and shipping hub in Asia since the 1980s. In 1998 the U.S. State Department complained that Taiwan's counter-narcotics program, while investigating more cases, seized fewer drugs and prosecuted fewer people.

In the past, Taiwan's drug factories produced large quantities of amphetamines. Aggressive Taiwanese police efforts, however, caused the producers to move their facilities to mainland China. About 68 percent of the methamphetamines and 42 percent of the heroin seized on Taiwan during the first eleven months of 1998 came from mainland China (Central Intelligence Agency, 2000b).

Proposed Solutions and Strategies

To prepare for the substance-abuse problems they will encounter when Hong Kong and Taiwan resume membership in the nation of China, officials, social planners, and representatives from antidrug committees in China need to explore ways in which to soften its harsh antidrug policy and shift the focus from punishment to prevention and treatment. If it does not make this shift in attitude, there well may come a time when the harsh, restrictive rules harm so many innocent Chinese directly or indirectly that the antidrug laws will be unenforced. To control successfully between 500,000 and a million Chinese drug addicts, using Mao's model, the Chinese government will need to take away what few rights the other two billion Chinese have only recently been able to wrench from the Communist Party. Many Chinese hold their few freedoms and rights dearly, as they should.

CONCLUSION

Certainly, it would be impossible to develop a worldview of substance abuse without having insight into the Chinese opium experience. The British showed that by flooding a market with a narcotic or drug that numbs the consciousness of the user, it is possible to addict large numbers of the disheartened and the hopeless in a disintegrating country. This same marketing strategy has been used by most mid-level and local pushers among the excluded and impoverished in the inner cities of Europe and the United States.

It is also important to have examined a case history of a prohibition model of drug control that worked. In this case, prohibition worked under a tight Communist regime where there were no or few individual freedoms. Would it work in other societies? For the Communist Chinese drug prohibition model to work in a democracy or even a semidemocracy, individual freedoms would have to be curtailed. Most would agree that to relinquish individual freedoms to stop illegal drug use would do more damage to the political and social structure of a society than the damage caused by illegal drug use.

REFERENCES

Associated Press. (1997, March 25). China orders crackdown on growing drug trade. New York: Author.

Central Intelligence Agency. (2000a). *The world factbook: Hong Kong.* Washington, D.C.: prepared by the Central Intelligence Agency for the use of U.S. Government officials. Retrieved November 14, 2000, from the World Wide Web: http://www.odci.gov/cia/publications/factbook/geos/fr.htm

Central Intelligence Agency. (2000b). *The world factbook: China.* Washington, D.C.: prepared by the Central Intelligence Agency for the use of U.S. Government officials. Retrieved November 14, 2000, from the World Wide Web: http://www.odci.gov/cia/publications/factbook/geos/fr.htm

Chinese Ministry of Health and UNAIDS Programme. (1997, November). *China Special Report: China Responds to AIDS.* Beijing: Author.

Dobson, C. (1992, October 4). The Hongkong connection: The declining use of opium in Hong Kong. *South China Morning Post,* p. 5. Retrieved November 12, 2000, from the World Wide Web from Lexis-Nexis.

DrugTexT Foundation. (1996). *The politics of heroin in Southeast Asia: China grows her own.* Amsterdam, The Netherlands: International Foundation on Drug Policy and Human Rights.

Encarta Desk Encyclopedia. (1998). China. Microsoft Corporation [CD-ROM].

Holley, D. (1990, July 23). Devil of opium addiction returns to prey on China. Los Angeles: Times Mirror, p. 1A.

Inglis, B. (1975). *The forbidden game.* New York: Charles Scribner's Sons.

Media Awareness Project. (2000). *China: China wrestles with drugs.* Melbourne, Australia: David Syme.

Ozanich, T. (1997, May 27). Treatment, executions designed to combat addiction. From correspondent Terry Ozanich. World Wide Web posted at 11:37 A.M. EDT.

Tho'Mas, K. (1997, July 10). Opium war: Britain stole Hong Kong from China. *Workers Worlds* (New York newspaper). Workers World Service. Retrieved October 28, 2000, from the World Wide Web: *http://workers.org*

United Nations, Economic and Social Council. (1951). *Offer for sale in Hong Kong of five hundred tons of opium at present in China.* New York.

Wu, Zunyou, Detels, R. and Jianpeng, Zhang. (1995, December). *Risk factors for intravenous drug use and sharing equipment among young male drug users in Southwest China.* Paper presented at the 1995 China International Symposium on AIDS, Beijing, China.

4

COLOMBIA

Andrew Cherry

INTRODUCTION

The only way to examine addiction and treatment using a global view is to look at the precursors to addiction: production, transport, and marketing. At the individual level, withdrawal, and overwhelming cravings are associated with drug addiction. At a political level, the money from illegal drugs is even more addictive and corrosive. Among countries that are considered the source of illegal drugs and the countries that are involved in trafficking illegal drugs, none are more ensnarled in this quasi-industry than Colombia in South America. Colombia is involved both as a source and as a trafficker. It is one of the primary drug source countries in South America and the world. It is also a major transport country. Not only are illegal drugs produced in Colombia smuggled north, but cocaine and heroin produced in other South American countries around the Andean region are shipped to Colombia and then smuggled north.

Drug Money–Ravaged Colombia

Since the 1980s, because of the illegal drug trade and subsequent drug war, Colombia has endured the worst human rights crisis in the Americas. The people of Colombia have faced the scourge of leftist insurgencies and right-wing death squads. Throughout the 1990s, as many as 3,000 civilians died from political violence each year. Many more were kidnapped and held for ransom (Marquez, 1997). In addition, at least 1.5 million people have been displaced since 1985, with more than 300,000 people displaced in 1998 and 2,945 people abducted in 1999 (Hall, 2000). In Colombia, *el narcotrafio* has filled morgues, spread addiction, turned schoolchildren into assassins, and made judges into martyrs.

Addiction in Colombia

In addition to the corruption of the political and economic systems, Colombia like all other source and trafficking countries has suffered a corresponding increase in drug addiction at all levels of society. There has also been an increase in drug-related crime, violence, and adolescent drug use.

The increase in Colombian drug use and addiction was not accidental. In many cases, addicting local people to cocaine was part of the plan to increase the profits from the illegal drug trade. One example of domestic addiction in Colombia that can be linked directly to the drug producers was the sudden and widespread addiction among Colombian youths in the early 1980s to *basuco* (coca paste). The first step in making cocaine is making coca paste. This product, which has many contaminates in it, is harmful when inhaled; it is also very addictive. Typically, *basuco* is smoked with marijuana or tobacco. *Basuco* was dumped on the Colombian illegal drug market by the cocaine producers because it was inexpensive to produce and the profits were reasonable. Because *basuco* was so cheap, it soon became more popular in many Colombian urban areas than marijuana. This phase of addiction in Colombia left thousands of addicts, many of whom suffer from permanent nervous disorders (Hanratty and Meditz, 1988). Yet, because so much of Colombia's resources are used to fight the revolutionary groups and the drug lords, the Colombian government has few resources to provide substance-abuse prevention and treatment. In fact, almost all alcohol and drug prevention and treatment programs in Colombia are nongovernmental. Private foundations, the United Nations, and the European Union are the primary funders of substance-abuse prevention and treatment in Colombia today (Pérez-Gómez, 1998).

One of the ironies about the drug abuse and addiction problem in Colombia is that for years officials in South America have maintained that there was not an addiction problem in developing countries like Colombia. Addiction was a problem found in rich countries, not poor countries. Unquestionably, there is some evidence to support this perception. Andean Indians have been chewing coca leaf for thousands of years to help them endure the thin air in the mountains and the rugged mountain life. When these coca leaf–chewing Indians came down from the mountains, they stopped chewing the leaf with few or no withdrawal problems. Unfortunately, the experiences of cocaine addicts today, in the urban areas of Colombia, have little in common with their Indian ancestors. The Colombian addicts have more in common with addicts worldwide who are physically and emotionally addicted to a substance that is illegal in most countries around the world (Montoya and Chilcoat, 1996).

Alcohol is the primary drug of use and abuse in Colombia. In several surveys made in treatment centers, it was determined that roughly 40 percent of the clients were treated for alcohol abuse, although most, about 85 percent, were polydrug users. However, although the number of alcoholics has remained fairly stable over the years, this is not true of the cocaine-addicted. The number of Colombians who use coca paste and cocaine has been increasing. In the mid-1980s, based on a national household survey, it was estimated that about 110,000 Colombians were using some form of cocaine. By the mid-1990s, surveys were discovering that more than 700,000 Colombians were using some form of cocaine (Pérez-Gómez, 1998).

Prevention and Drug Treatment

Drug abuse among Colombians became a growing problem in the mid-1970s, but it was not the focus of much attention until the mid-1980s. Colombia as a nation, its culture, and its infrastructure have been in a permanent state of deterioration since the 1980s. Such a state of anomie could be contributing to the increase in drug use.

Although all of the drug-treatment centers and clinics are supposed to be members of the Colombian Drug Treatment Network, which is under the Ministry of Health, participation among these centers is poor. The network is supposed to maintain records of the number of addicts being treated and outcome data, but it lacks adequate financial support, experienced personnel, and the operational authority to exert adequate control over the large number of heterogeneous drug-treatment institutions. Thus, the extent of the drug problem and the incident rates of addiction in Colombia must be extrapolated from surveys of regions of the country and the data kept by treatment centers. Some clinicians and advocates of drug treatment suspect that the number of cases and descriptive data on those treated are not collected in a serious and scientific way because there is no interest at the government level in knowing the parameters of the addicted population (Pérez-Gómez, 1998).

A Brief Profile of Colombia

The relationship between the United States and Colombia was first tested with land disputes during the construction of the Panama Canal. The gold rush in California made it clear that a canal through Central America which linked the Atlantic and Pacific Oceans was needed. In 1899 the U.S. Congress created the Isthmian Canal Commission to undertake the task. Shortly afterward, the United States obtained a strip of land six miles (9.5 kilometers) wide across the Isthmus of Panama; however, the Colombian Senate refused to ratify the lease.

In 1903 Panamanian rebels, backed by the U.S. government, rebelled against Colombia and declared Panama to be a free and separate country from Colombia. The rebel leaders then signed the Hay-Bunau-Varilla Treaty, which gave the United States a secured and perpetual lease on a ten-mile (16-kilometer) strip for the canal. In return, the United States guaranteed the independence of Panama. In 1907 the U.S. Army Corps of Engineers began construction, and the canal opened in 1914. The construction cost of the canal was $335 million (Bushnell, 1993).

Even after this land grab by the United States, Colombia still has coasts on both the Caribbean Sea and the Pacific Ocean. The mainland territory can be divided into four major geographical regions: the Andean highlands (composed of three mountain ranges and intervening valley lowlands), the Caribbean lowlands, the Pacific lowlands, and the tropical rain forest of eastern Colombia.

While there is a wide variation in temperature across Colombia, there is little seasonal change. Rather, the climate of a region is determined by its elevation. The temperature variations consist of hot regions in the country (areas under 900 meters [2,952 ft.] above sea level), temperate regions (areas between 900 and 1,980 meters [2,952–6,495 ft.]), and cold regions (areas from 1,980 meters to about 3,500 meters [6,495–11,484] above sea level). Precipitation is generally moderate to heavy, with the highest levels of rain occurring in the Pacific lowlands and in the Caribbean regions of eastern Colombia (Hanratty and Meditz, 1988). This variation in temperature and altitude permits the cultivation of coca, which needs a mountainous altitude, and poppies, which are grown at a much lower altitude.

Approximately 40 million people live in Colombia. It has a growth rate of about 2 percent annually. In urban areas, about 90 percent of Colombian children between the ages of seven and eleven attend primary school; in rural areas, it is close to 70 percent. In the more isolated communities, fewer than 50 percent of the children may be attending primary school. About 30 percent of those twelve years of age or older attend secondary school. Even so, Colombian officials estimate that 88 percent of Colombians are literate (Hanratty and Meditz, 1988).

Health care and medical services, which improved in the 1970s and 1980s, still left the rural and urban poor suffering from higher mortality (death) and morbidity (disease rates). In 1988 the life expectancy at birth was estimated to be sixty-eight years for females and sixty-four years for males (Hanratty and Meditz, 1988).

Spanish is the official language of Colombia. The population is made up primarily of five ethnic groups: mestizos, 50 percent; whites, 25 percent; mulattoes and zambos (black-Indian mix), 20 percent; blacks, 4 percent; and Indians, 1 percent (Hanratty and Meditz, 1988).

The Concordat of 1973 (a formal agreement between the pope of the Catholic Church and a national government concerning religious affairs in a country) preserved the privileged status of the Roman Catholic Church over other religious groups. More than 95 percent of the people of Colombia are Roman Catholic; the remainder belong primarily to various Protestant groups (Hanratty and Meditz, 1988).

The gross domestic product (GDP) is approximately $35 billion (U.S. currency). The per capita income is roughly $875 (U.S. currency) per year. The primary legal export crops are coffee, bananas, cut flowers, sugarcane, and cotton (Hanratty and Meditz, 1988).

Colombia is rich in many natural resources. It has large deposits of precious metals including gold, platinum, and silver. Colombia also has one of the few known deposits of emeralds in the world. Colombia has Latin America's largest coal reserve and large deposits of oil and natural gas. The exploitation of Colombia's oil resources by multinational corporations is at the heart of one rebel group's reason for fighting in the civil war (Hanratty and Meditz, 1988).

The Social Structure

Although Colombia is the oldest democracy in South America, a privileged class rules the country. Colombia's social structure is based on the Spanish colonial and postindependence periods. Spanish authorities established a highly stratified social system in colonial Colombia, then called New Granada. *Peninsulares*, persons of Spanish descent (persons born in Spain) controlled the colony. Under the *peninsulares* were the *criollos*, those of Spanish descent but born in New Granada. Mestizos constituted the lower stratum of society. Mulattoes, zambos (black-Indian mix), and blacks existed at the margin of colonial society. Indians were not included in Colombian colonial society. After independence, the *criollos* took control of the country away from the *peninsulares*. The mixed-race citizens gained a modicum of social mobility; however, it was granted to individuals not to groups (Hanratty and Meditz, 1988).

The control of political power in Colombia continues to be in the hands of the upper class. Although it makes up only 5 percent of the population, the upper class dominates the nation's economic and political institutions. The upper class, which includes both traditional large landowners with distinguished family lineages and major entrepreneurs, considers itself to be the keepers of the nation's cultural heritage. The middle class makes up 20 percent of the population (Hanratty and Meditz, 1988).

In the latter part of the twentieth century, the relatively stable political environment allowed for sustained economic growth. This in turn resulted in major social changes. The development of industry in Bogotá, Cali, Medellín, and Barranquilla provided high paying jobs which in turn caused a mass migration of the rural poor into these industrial centers from the countryside. By the early 1980s, approximately 70 percent of all Colombians lived in urban areas, one of the highest rates in Latin America. This urbanization, however, also weakened kinship ties and often destroyed the extended family structure (Hanratty and Meditz, 1988). Without the support of extended families, the rural poor who moved to the cities were more susceptible to drug use and addiction than before.

The Civil War in Colombia

To understand the dynamics of illegal drugs in Colombia, one needs to have some understanding of the role of the revolutionary groups. In the 1960s Communist insurgents spread across Central and South America trying, and succeeding sometimes, to overthrow established authority. In Colombia it started with rebels fighting for the rights of poor peasants who suffered from extreme poverty, governmental neglect, exclusion, and abuse from right-wing paramilitary groups and rebels (*Encarta Desk Encyclopedia*, 1998). In Colombia, four major revolutionary groups have fought in the civil war since 1960: the Revolutionary Armed Forces of Colombia (Fuerzas Armadas Revolucionarias de Colombia, or FARC), the National Liberation Army (Ejército de Liberación Nacional, or ELN), the Popular Liberation Army (Ejército Popular de Liberación, or EPL), and the 19th of April Movement (Movimiento 19 de Abril, or M-19). Other, smaller guerrilla groups have also participated (Hanratty and Meditz, 1988).

Both the revolutionary groups and the paramilitary groups target civilians who they believe support the other side. The revolutionary groups are responsible for the majority of kidnappings for profit; the paramilitary groups are responsible for most of the terrorist murders and most of the massive displacement of the rural poor.

The Colombian army, which itself is directly responsible for many of the human rights violations, has extensive links to right-wing paramilitary forces at the local and regional levels. Some army officers have directly assisted the paramilitary groups in terrorist acts; others have closed their eyes to paramilitary acts of violence and murder (*Encarta Desk Encyclopedia*, 1998).

The ELN is attempting to force the government to nationalize the petroleum industry and terminate all oil-exploration contracts with multinational firms. To this end, between January 1988 and June 2000, the ELN carried out over 400 attacks on Colombia's largest oil pipeline (Bushnell, 1993).

After forty years of fighting, on October 24, 1999, some 10 million Colombians, 25 percent of the population, in all parts of Colombia marched for peace. They were demonstrating their support for a negotiated solution to the conflict and an end to the violence from all sides (Latin America Working Group, 1999).

At the same time, the United States was increasing the amount of money available to fight the drug war in Colombia. In 1997 U.S. aid to Colombia was approximately $95 million (U.S. currency). In 1999, it was $289 million. In 2000, the U.S. Congress appropriated $1.3 billion in emergency assistance for fighting the illegal drug trade in Colombia.

According to some, the money to fight drug production in Colombia has contributed to the increase in the international illegal drug trade and is partly responsible for destabilizing the Colombian government. The tremendous amount of illegal drug money in Colombia is rivaled only by the sums of money involved in fighting cultivation and production in Colombia.

Stopping the flow of drugs into the United States has proven to be more difficult than one would think. Complicating the issue in Colombia is the civil war. The illegal drug trade has become intertwined with the forty-year-old civil war being fought against the Colombian government. For this reason, many Colombian officials, other leaders in South America, and many in the United States have warned that the millions of dollars from the United States earmarked for drug eradication in Colombia have instead been used to fight revolutionaries. The fear is that this use of U.S. drug eradication dollars will drive the Colombian revolutionaries into other countries in South America and thus spread the civil war into nations on Colombia's borders (Hall, 2000).

Furthermore, part of the $1.3 billion package was to be used to support sending U.S. troops to Colombia to train Colombian soldiers and to help eradicate drug crops. Not unexpectedly, in the United States, there were cries of Colombia's becoming another Vietnam. Although the number of U.S. soldiers who were going to Colombia was small, the fear of many political leaders in the United States and other countries in the Andean region was that this was only the beginning of a U.S. military intervention. Once the precedent was set, more troops and military equipment would be sent to fight the drug growers and wind up in the hands of the right-wing paramilitary groups.

While the Colombian civil war is complicated and rests on divergent political ideologies, in terms of drug cultivation and production the issue is simple. When peasant farmers grow illegal drug crops, rebel groups protect the crops from the Colombian right-wing paramilitary groups that attempt to destroy it. For protection, the farmers pay a tax to the rebels. After the farmer sells the raw materials to producers, right-wing militant groups protect the manufacturers and the traffickers from revolutionaries, the military, and each other.

Revolutionaries profit by taxing the drug trade in areas they control. Paramilitary groups are directly tied to the drug traffickers. In addition, paramilitary groups run a secret war, assassinating intellectuals and human rights defenders who speak out against them. By giving interdiction money to the

Colombian military, it is said, the United States is aiding the right-wing paramilitary groups.

VIGNETTE

Alberto Velazco, a forty-one-year-old Guambiare Indian, was a small farmer who grew poppies in the mountains outside Popayan (a city in southwest Colombia, located south of Cali, founded in 1536). Mr. Velazco said that agents who wanted his neighbors and him to grow illegal drug plants came to his community after a plant fungus disease ruined the tribe's potato and onion crops. Mr. Velazco said that the first illegal drug agent was a North American. For the farmers who agreed to grow poppies, the drug agent supplied seeds, fertilizer, and four months' worth of groceries, and he pledged to buy the opium harvest for a set price.

"It started out with only a few people growing opium poppies," said the tribal chief. "After that, poppy flowers started appearing everywhere." In a short period, 70 percent of the 13,500 Guambiare had given up raising food crops and were growing poppies, cutting down virgin forests to do so (Schemo, 1998a). However, just like the Colombians living in the highlands and growing coca, the Guambiare saw their society change in profound ways. Their respect for nature was the first to fall. Family members and tribal leaders were at odds over how to deal with the influx of money, strangers, and violence. Finally, tribal leaders realized that the drug money was destroying their community. They convinced the tribe membership to reclaim their traditions and their ancestral way of life. Tribal leaders presented the government their "Plan of Life" to help the Guambiare give up poppy cultivation. It was not easy. Some tribesmen even threatened the leader's life, and a letter purporting to be from the local revolutionary group warned the tribe not to stop growing poppies.

The tribe responded to the threat by going to the revolutionary commander and explaining their Plan of Life. After the meeting, the commander pledged not to interfere in the tribe's switch to legal crops. Although U.S. officials maintain that crop-substitution efforts will not work in Colombia because the rebels will not let the peasants stop growing coca and poppies, Juan Carlos Palou, the director of Plante, Colombia's crop-substitution program, said in 1998 that no farmer had ever been killed by rebels for giving up cultivation of illicit crops (Schemo, 1998a).

OVERVIEW OF ADDICTION AND BASIC DEMOGRAPHICS

Colombia has the most liberal drug laws in the Americas. Possession of small quantities of all drugs is legal. Drugs intended for personal use are permitted as a *personal dose*. A personal dose of marijuana is 20 grams.

Although alcohol is the most widely abused drug in Colombia, the primary illegal drugs used are marijuana, *basuco*, and cocaine. Over the years, there has been real concern and interest in how the widespread availability and easy access to cheap cocaine derivatives such as *basuco* would affect the number of people who use cocaine or a derivative. The question was, "Would easy access to cheap cocaine tend to increase addiction?" By the mid-1990s, it was becoming evident that the cocaine problem was continuing to increase in Colombia. In the United States, after reaching a peak in the early 1990s, the use of cocaine began to decline. At the same time, it continued to increase markedly in Colombia, somewhat offsetting the reduced demand in the United States (Montoya and Chilcoat, 1996). Based on a survey made of households, between the mid-1980s and the mid-1990s, the number of people who used or had a history of drug use went up threefold. Although high, this may be an undercount. In another study, 4 percent of those surveyed had used some form of cocaine in the past month (Montoya and Chilcoat, 1996). If these percentages held true nationally, by extrapolation, there would be 1,600,000 regular users of a cocaine derivative in Colombia out of a nation of 40 million.

HISTORY OF DRUG USE IN COLOMBIA

Many of the naturally occurring drugs that are used in the world today with the exception of alcohol, opium, and marijuana came from South America. Coffee, tobacco, cocoa (chocolate), and coca (cocaine) were known only in the Americas before the voyages of Christopher Columbus. The Inca used the coca leaf in virtually all religious rituals and state ceremonies. All Inca noblemen were buried with a plentiful supply of coca leaf. Few Spanish conquistadors chewed the coca leaf because of superstition. Even so, they controlled the coca leaf supply and gave it to the Indians because when chewing coca leaf, the Indians worked harder on less food (Brecher, 1972).

Historically, the cultivation of the coca shrub has played an important role in Andean society from pre-Columbian times to the present. Nevertheless, the rapid expansion of commercial and illegal coca cultivation in the early 1980s in areas that are outside of the traditional coca-growing regions of the Andes, such as the Bolivian Yungas, owe their expansion not to pre-Columbian tradition but to the increased world demand for cocaine, particularly in the United States and Western Europe (Ivins, 1999).

The money involved in the international illegal drug trade is exceeded only by that in the world's arms trade. As might be expected, both are intertwined in the spread of drug addiction and AIDS through national terrorism and guerrilla warfare.

Coca/Cocaine Production and Trafficking

The coca plant is grown only in the Andean region of South America, primarily in Bolivia and Peru. At some collection points, a simple industrial product, coca paste (cocaine sulfate), is also produced. The buyers of the coca leaf and coca paste, the producers of powder cocaine, and those involved in trafficking are almost exclusively Colombians. The manufacturing and transport, as well as the wholesale distribution, of cocaine in the United States are controlled by Colombians (Ivins, 1999).

Bolivia and Peru have also experienced the effect of the drug money boom. The influx of large amounts of drug money attracted small family farmers into the high-risk business of growing coca leaf. Even so, few farmers became rich.

Colombia Peasant Farmers and Drug Cultivation

For struggling rural farmers, the decision to grow coca or poppy was a practical one. There was no legitimate way to earn a living, and drug crops offered an income that was unheard of since the heyday of skyrocketing coffee prices in the early 1970s. Peasant farmers (called *cocaleros* when they grow coca) who climbed on the coca bandwagon early enjoyed five years of prosperity referred to as *La Bonanza*. Nonetheless, as more peasant farmers grew coca rather than food crops, prices for coca leaf dropped and the cost of the food rose. Additionally, it became harder to harvest a coca crop. Crop-dusting planes, financed by the U.S. antidrug program, poisoned the fields from the air and soldiers destroyed them on the ground.

As life in these rural communities began to unravel, the coca farmers discovered that, although Colombia was spending $1.1 billion a year fighting drug trafficking, and the U.S. government tripled funding for Colombia's antinarcotics police and military, there was little or no money available to help them grow legal crops (Schemo, 1998b). Furthermore, during this period, U.S. officials at the Bank for Inter-American Development voted against a $90 million loan to increase crop substitution in Colombia, according to a report made by the Washington Office on Latin America (Schemo, 1998b).

Abuse and exploitation of the peasants by the army, drug lords, paramilitary units, and revolutionary groups have weakened the traditional ties of the peasants to the land. Civil strife—the army and landowner-financed paramilitary groups fighting against leftist revolutionaries—and the purchase of vast tracts of farmland by drug lords have left an estimated 1.2 million Colombians landless. Since moving toward a market economy in the early 1990s, thousands of small farmers in Colombia have gone out of business, unable to compete with the world prices for corn, rice, and other grains. Although many farm families have migrated to urban areas, other farmers moved to remote areas of Colombia to grow coca. The lack of roads to these remote areas is an advantage for the coca growers. The military and right-wing groups cannot get to their fields. Coca and poppy buyers fly into clandestine airstrips to purchase the crops.

The U.S. Drug War in Colombia

A major focus of the U.S. government's strategy to reduce drug use and addiction in the United States was to eradicate the coca and opium fields in Colombia and destroy the labs that manufacture the final product. The focus on Colombia makes sense at some level, especially when 80 percent of the cocaine sold in the United States has been coming from Colombia. The question, however, that needed to be asked was related to the approach. Was a U.S. military eradication program the best approach for reducing coca and poppy farming in Colombia? Or, would crop substitution work better? Until now, a crop-substitution strategy has not been an option in Colombia because a great deal of the Colombian land used to produce coca and poppy is in the hands of rebel groups. Neither the Colombian government nor the United States wants to give aid to rebel groups in the form of crop-substitution money (Schemo, 1998a).

The impact of the eradication program was mixed. In 1997 Colombian military pilots sprayed herbicides on 100,000 hectares (40,000 acres) of coca crops. To compensate for their loss, farmers increased the total area under coca cultivation by 20 percent. Consequently, although about 54,000 hectares of coca plants were destroyed and tens of thousands of tons of cocaine and heroin were seized between 1988 and 1995, it had "little impact on the availability of illegal drugs in the United States," according to a 1997 report published by the General Accounting Office (Schemo, 1998b).

Controlling Chemicals Used in Drug Production

Another side to the illicit drug industry is the legal commercial chemical industry and the legal chemicals needed to process such raw materials as coca paste and raw opium into cocaine and heroin. These commercially produced, available chemicals are also used in the illegal manufacture of synthetic drugs (designer drugs), including methamphetamine (ICE), phencyclidine (PCP), and Ecstasy. These synthetic drugs are referred to as designer drugs because they use the chemical analog (or chemical formula) of a controlled substance such as cocaine. The synthetic chemical structure is designed to be similar to a controlled substance (e.g., cocaine) and to produce a similar effect in humans when consumed. Chemicals used in the processing or production of illegal drugs are known as precursors to drug production (Monastero, 1985).

Chemicals are used to dissolve solid raw materials, to dilute mixtures, to separate compounds, and to purify the final product—the consumed drug. A precursor for cocaine is the coca leaf, a reagent is sulfuric acid, and a solvent used in the manufacturing process is acetone. For methamphetamine, a precursor is phenyl-2-propanone, a reagent is sulfuric acid, and a solvent is methanol. Many of these chemicals, used to produce or refine illicit drugs, are also used in industry to produce a myriad of items, and these legal items are produced in tremendous quantities. Acetone, for instance, is used as a solvent in processing opium and coca leaves; however, it is also used to make paints, lubricants, pharmaceuticals, cosmetics, and agricultural products.

Some industrial chemicals have been regulated for years. Piperidine, a precursor to the production of PCP, is subject to reporting requirements under U.S. law as stipulated in the Controlled Substances Act. As a direct result of this law, in the first fifteen years of its existence, the Drug Enforcement Agency seized four clandestine PCP laboratories and located ten operations that received chemicals from legitimate channels by posing as legitimate businesses (Monastero, 1985).

Using Fungus to Kill Coca Plants and Poppies

Spraying herbicide on crops of illegal drugs became an eradication strategy used by the United States in the war on drugs in Mexico in the 1970s. The problem with spraying herbicides to eradicate poppy fields, however, is that ninety days after spraying and destroying a poppy field, the same field can be back in production. For this and other reasons, the U.S. government adopted a program to spray a deadly fungus on the coca plants and poppy fields in Colombia. This fungus does not just kill the plant, it infects the soil of the fields and renders the fields useless for farming. The basic flaw in this strategy is that if the eradication program succeeds, drugs will simply be grown, processed, and shipped into the United States from other countries. As long as there is a strong demand for illegal drugs in the United States and Western Europe, there will be a means to supply them.

International environmentalists are very concerned about the impact on the environment when large tracks of farmland are sprayed with the coca fungus, *fusarium oxysporum*. There is little scientific data about how this fungus will affect an area's ecosystem. Although U.S. officials insist that the fungus be sprayed on the Colombian drug crops, environmentalists in Florida blocked testing of a similar fungus on marijuana fields in Florida because of the fear it would kill more than the marijuana.

Colombia has its own doubts about the coca fungus. Its environmental minister at the time, Juan Mayr, insisted that tests of the fungus be conducted outside Colombia. He feared that the fungus could hold "grave risks to the environment and human health" ("Toxic War," 2000).

How Colombia Became the Illicit Drug Capital of the World

Over the last half of the twentieth century, the United States funded and conducted numerous eradication and interdiction programs, yet not one program succeeded in reducing the supply of illegal drugs in the United

States. Indeed, for the most part, these interdiction and eradication programs actually increased the drug supply and thus addiction. Eradication programs paid for by the U.S. government drove drug producers into new countries and regions. Interdiction efforts backed by the United States resulted in the development of new smuggling routes through new countries and the introduction of or widespread availability of new, highly addictive drugs.

When heroin became widespread in U.S. cities (via the supply route called the "French connection"), elected officials believed that by destroying the Turkey–France–United States heroin supply line, they would destroy heroin trafficking and reduce addiction in the United States. Despite the success in breaking the French connection, heroin production simply moved from Turkey to Mexico and Asia. The Mexican and Southeast Asian poppy growers and heroin producers continued to be major producers of heroin into the twenty-first century. Although, in the United States, Turkey was no longer the primary source of heroin, Turkey and other Eastern European countries continued to supply much of the heroin used in Western Europe (Zeese, 2000).

President Richard Nixon's first drug war campaign, called Operation Intercept, targeted smugglers bringing illegal drugs to the United States across the Mexican-American border. The plan called for searching every third vehicle crossing the Mexican border into the United States. Drug traffickers simply switched from smuggling drugs across the Mexican border to using boats and planes. The Mexican border interdiction effort also expanded the sale of heroin from Southeast Asia. It had gained a foothold in the U.S. drug market during the Vietnam War (Zeese, 2000).

In the end, the border searches so disrupted commerce between the United States and Mexico it could not be sustained. By the time the Nixon program ended, Mexican traffickers not only had land routes across the Mexican-American border, but also sea and air routes to move the illegal drugs.

The paraquat spraying program in Mexico in the 1970s (used after the failure of Operation Intercept) had a similar disastrous outcome. Paraquat, a herbicide, was sprayed on marijuana and poppy fields in Mexico in an attempt to eradicate the marijuana and poppy plants being grown by small Mexican farmers. Paraquat-tainted marijuana from Mexico caused a scare among marijuana users in the United States, which drove up the price and increased the growing of domestic marijuana in the United States. By the end of the twentieth century, domestically grown marijuana accounted for roughly 25 percent of all marijuana consumed in the United States. In addition, the Colombian marijuana trade was born. No longer satisfied with supplying Mexican traffickers with marijuana, Colombian traffickers began shipping their own bales of marijuana directly to the United States, using their own smuggling routes (Zeese, 2000).

Previous failures, however, did not deter U.S. politicians. President Ronald Reagan's Florida interdiction program, in the early 1980s, was another spectacular failure. At the time, almost all of the Colombian marijuana went through South Florida. Miami had the largest Colombian population in the United States, so it was easy for the drug traffickers to integrate into the community. To stop the influx of Colombian marijuana, President Reagan escalated the interdiction effort by using the military to stop the flood of Colombian marijuana from coming into the United States.

The results were consistent with past interdiction efforts. Colombian traffickers realized they would be caught less often and make a larger profit if they switched from marijuana to the less bulky cocaine. The traffickers also developed new smuggling routes along the west and gulf coasts of the United States and through Mexico. This interdiction effort resulted in an increase in the purity of cocaine, a decrease in price, a steady supply, and soaring cocaine addiction problems in the United States, Colombia, Mexico, and other countries involved in smuggling cocaine into the United States (Zeese, 2000).

President George H.W. Bush had his own solution to the overwhelming cocaine problem that developed in the United States after Reagan's Florida interdiction program. The Bush plan was to increase military and other law enforcement efforts in the Andean region to stop cocaine production at its source. His program did not reduce the supply of coca leaf to the drug producers. It did manage, however, to force large farmers to franchise out the growing of coca plants (a very hardy plant) and poppy plants to small farmers who were always struggling to earn a living for their families. Consequently, the cocaine producers are still there, and the supply of coca leaf is still abundant (Zeese, 2000).

While the Andean eradication efforts were in full swing, President Bush's interdiction effort focused on drug trafficking and money laundering in Panama. The money-laundering enterprise in Panama was protected by the president of Panama, Manuel Noriega. President Bush ordered an invasion of Panama to arrest Noriega. The invasion was successful. Noriega was taken to the United States where he stood trial and was found guilty and sentenced to forty years in a U.S. federal prison. This solved the Noriega problem, but it did not slow the flow of illegal drugs into the United States. The drug traffickers simply moved their operations into other Central American countries and the Caribbean Islands. Moreover, they became more sophisticated in the smuggling trade and in their money-laundering activities (Zeese, 2000).

The U.S. banking and tax laws require the filing of reports on currency transactions exceeding $10,000. Traffickers trying to hide illicit drug money have evaded U.S. reporting rules by smuggling the cash out of the United States. Afterward, the money is deposited in foreign financial institutions. This approach makes the money more difficult to trace, and the money can be spent or transferred back to the United States or other countries with less risk of exposure. By the end of the twentieth century, U.S. Treasury Department and Customs Service officials estimated that the amount of currency being smuggled out of the United States was in the billions of dollars each year (U.S. Senate, 1994).

The Peruvian shoot-down strategy, conducted during the early years of the Clinton administration, was another program that escalated the war against drugs. The United States provided intelligence to the Peruvian military so they could shoot down airplanes suspected of transporting coca paste from growers in Peru to cocaine producers in Colombia. This policy resulted in decreasing the coca coming from the traditional coca regions of Peru and Bolivia and increasing the number of new coca farmers in Colombia to fill the gap (Zeese, 2000). On April 20, 2001, the policy also resulted in the death of a missionary and her seven-month-old adopted daughter from Michigan who were in a plane carrying missionaries over the Amazon river. A U.S. radar plane guided the Peruvian A-37 military jet in for the kill. The missionaries' plane was mistaken for a drug-smuggling flight. After the shoot-down, the U.S. Central Intelligence Agency grounded its anti-drug mission over Colombia and Peru (Rosenberg, 2001).

Clinton's Colombian eradication program continued the long history of failed U.S. interdiction and eradication policies. Colombia has been the site of the most aggressive herbicide-spraying programs in the world, and it has been the largest recipient of military aid from the United States outside of the Middle East. Despite these efforts, illegal drug production and trafficking, rather than declining, has increased in Colombia. The reaction from Washington was to escalate the war on drugs once again. In the year 2000, Congress appropriated $1.3 billion to expand the drug war in Colombia (Zeese, 2000). It takes several years to see what changes in the drug trade will result from the latest infusion of dollars into the U.S. war on drugs, but expectations are low. The question was, will the additional $1.3 billion be more effective in reducing the U.S. drug problem than the first $250 billion spent on the drug war? One effect of the forty-year drug war, which cannot be disputed, is that Colombia went from a major coffee-producing country to the undisputed illegal drug capital of the world.

The Influence of Illegal Drugs on Colombia

Although there is little government interest in drug addiction treatment in Colombia, there is a great deal of government interest in the money involved in the illegal drug trade. The enormous amount of money generated by drug trafficking nearly overwhelms Colombia's national economy, or at the very least dwarfs the earnings from most traditional and legal commodity exports. Because of political corruption, paid for with illegal drug money, Colombia has experienced the partial collapse of certain state functions, such as the administration of justice and the control of public order. The Colombian people, particularly Colombian politicians, have come to view narco-terrorism as the principal problem, not drug trafficking (Marquez, 1997).

Colombian officials, however, face a perplexing dilemma: How do they reduce narco-terrorism while, at the same time, capturing the economic benefits from drug trafficking? The huge inflow of foreign currency into Colombia has created a strong incentive for the Colombian government to develop policies to seize as much of the illegal drug money as possible. While the Colombian government is fighting a war against narco-terrorists, they continue to institutionalize programs to net even larger sums of drug money by setting up trading windows at the Central Bank of Colombia for the repatriation (laundering) of foreign capital. They also have regular tax amnesties which, among other benefits, legalize illicit profits (U.S. Senate, 1994).

Colombian Financial Infrastructure and the Illegal Drug Business

In fact, without the economic and financial infrastructure, the Colombian illegal drug trade could not have grown so rapidly or become so widespread. Despite the illegal nature of the drug trade, the financial sector of Colombia successfully adapted and developed channels to blend the large sums of drug revenues into the country's mainstream financial sector. Indeed, because of the modern financial services available in Colombia in the 1970s, which provided an easy way to launder drug money, both drug trafficking and the major drug cartels could be financed. Today, legal and illegal monies and business practices are so intertwined it is impossible to tell where the traditional form of economic wealth ends and the new drug money begins. By the end of the twentieth century, the drug traffickers were fully integrated into the Colombian economy.

Narco-Investment in Colombia

There is another perception about Colombian drug traffickers that needs to be cleared up before one can understand the detrimental nature of such large sums of illegal drug money coming into a country. The Colombian drug lords have not just squandered their wealth on unproductive luxury goods, as is popularly believed; they have invested their ill-gotten wealth throughout Colombia. This, in combination with the wide availability of U.S. dollars and the dollarization of the Colombian economy, has meant that Colombia was able to avoid the drastic devaluation in the currency and hyperinflation that occurred elsewhere in Latin America. The official exchange rate and the black market rate for dollars have been about equal since the mid-1980s. At times, the official Colombian bank rate for U.S. dollars is even higher than the black market rate. This illustrates how much hard currency (U.S. dollars) is circulating in Colombia's economy. This illegal drug money has been invested in legitimate industry, retailing, and communications. It is now providing a legitimate source of money for the drug cartels.

Although narco-investments can be found throughout Colombia, the most obvious large investments have been made in the countryside. There has been a major turnover of land from the peasants and the traditional Colombian landowners to drug cartels and drug lords. It is estimated that there are 13 million hectares (1 hectare equals 2.5 acres) under cultivation in Colombia; drug dealers control approximately 3 million hectares of this land. To put that in historical perspective, Colombia has had a land reform program for about twenty-five years. The state has distributed 900,000 hectares to landless people. In the 1980s so much of the land was bought by drug dealers that it became a "counter–land reform," with three times the land passing into the hands of the drug loads as the peasants.

Dismantling the Cali Cocaine Cartels

As demand for marijuana and later cocaine increased in the United States, criminal syndicates in Colombia quickly formed to help meet the U.S. demand. By the 1980s and 1990s, Colombian democracy was, for all intents and purposes, in the hands of the major cocaine-trafficking cartels based in Medellín and Cali.

The cartels used their illegal drug money to corrupt judges and politicians with huge payoffs. Public officials who could not be bribed where intimidated or killed by hired assassins known as *sicarios*. The drug lords also developed ties with various right-wing paramilitary groups. These paramilitary groups were responsible for systematically killing leftist politicians and their supporters in the 1980s. Over the years, paramilitary groups have allegedly murdered several hundred public officials who opposed them (Hall, 2000).

Not only did the drug lords hire and support dangerous right-wing paramilitary groups, the drug lords were dangerous in their own right. For example, Pablo Escobar Gavíria, a very powerful drug kingpin, is suspected of having a Colombian passenger airplane blown up because he wanted two people on the airplane killed. Altogether, 107 passengers died.

At the same time, Pablo Escobar and other drug lords were trying to improve their images among the poor of Colombia. Escobar, for instance, handed out cash to the urban poor, built low-income housing in the slums, purchased sports teams, and constructed sports stadiums. In 1982 Escobar was elected as an alternate congressional representative on a Liberal Party slate (a political party supported by Colombian drug lords) in his home department of Antioquia (Hanratty and Meditz, 1988). When Escobar was killed in a shoot-out while on the run from police, others quickly filled the gap he left, and the tons of cocaine being smuggled into the United States did not miss a beat.

SUBSTANCE ABUSE IN COLOMBIA TODAY

Political Views and Public Policies

Treatment for addiction has a low priority in Colombia. Officials in Colombia rightly point out that there are health issues and concerns that are more important or at least as important as drug treatment. They cannot see reducing prenatal care and vaccination programs for innocent children to increase drug treatment beds for drug addicts. The Colombian people, however, were more troubled by the increase in alcohol and drug addiction than were their elected officials. By 1990 surveys conducted of the Colombian public discovered that drug use had become a serious public concern following street violence, guerrillas, narco-trafficking, kidnapping, and unemployment (Hall, 2000). This result suggests that the average Colombian's view of drug use was that it was not only widespread but also creating problems for a lot of people who were not using drugs. As a result of the governmental lack of interest, statistics on incidents are sparse and often vary with the person or group conducting the study. Government-sponsored studies tend to find fewer addicts than studies funded by organizations outside of the Colombian government.

The Government Provides Some Residential Treatment Beds

The Colombian government, consistent with its lack of interest in addiction treatment, funds only 200 substance-abuse beds in all of Colombia. These beds, located in several mental hospitals, are typically filled with mental patients.

The lack of government involvement in treating addiction does not mean, however, that no substance-abuse treatment is available in Colombia. More than 150 private, nongovernment drug-treatment centers in Colombia provide some degree of service to as many as 20,000 drug-addicted people each year.

Social Views, Customs, and Drug Treatment Practices

The current Colombian models for treating drug addiction began with the therapeutic community model, for example, Daytop Village and Phoenix House, used in North America and Europe. The confrontational approach, which is an integral part of the therapeutic community model in the United States for the most part, was dropped from the Colombian model. The confrontational approach drove many Colombian addicts away from treatment. Today, these Colombian treatment centers use a modified or "softer" version of this approach. These centers also include Alcoholics Anonymous (AA) or Narcotics Anonymous (NA) as support systems, particularly after treatment. These Colombian AAs and NAs function in much the same way as traditional AAs and NAs function in the United States. By the end of the twentieth century, there were over 200 AA groups in Colombia; however, there were less than a dozen functioning NA groups.

Up until the 1980s, the only treatment available for addiction was at a mental hospital. Needless to say, rather than go to a mental hospital, many opted for no treatment. Today, private and nonprofit drug-treatment centers provide various types of treatment such as short-term residential, nonresidential day treatment, and outpatient centers.

Colombian clinicians who treat addiction and the general public at large tend to believe that the addicted are responsible for a large part of their addiction, particularly drug addicts. They point out that no one is forced to become an addict, and understanding the underlying reasons for an individual's drug use does not rule out self-responsibility. The objectives of treatment are the development of self-control, including the avoidance of situations and circumstances that may trigger relapse (Pérez-Gómez, 1998).

Compared to U.S. drug-treatment centers, Colombian drug-treatment centers tend to be less rigid in demanding total abstinence from clients, especially in the beginning phase of treatment. This reduced emphasis on total abstinence is consistent with the philosophy underlying treatment— addiction is regarded as a social problem.

Colombian leaders in addiction treatment have rejected the medical model as the explanation of addiction. As such, drug abuse is not considered a disease, and drug users are not considered sick people. Even so, clinicians agree that addiction harms the individual, the family, and the community.

THE FUTURE OF DRUG TREATMENT IN COLOMBIA

A concerted effort is needed to develop national prevention programs to reduce the number of young addicts (fourteen to sixteen years of age) and of girls who are becoming involved in drugs in ever-growing numbers. Programming must be developed to deal with the changing drug scene. Many teenagers have begun to use benzodiazepines and Rohypnol, and a growing number of adolescents are using heroin.

There is concern in Colombia, and in the international drug-treatment community, about the increase in heroin production in Colombia. If it follows modern trends, the more production there is, the more people will use heroin. If there is also a corresponding increase in intravenous heroin use, then one must anticipate an increase in HIV/AIDS infections. At the end of the twentieth century, official reports listed homosexual intercourse as the cause of 80 percent of HIV infections in Colombia. Drug abuse was not listed among the causes of HIV in Colombia in 1996 (Ministerio de Salud, 1996).

The possibility that heroin addiction will spread and alcohol and cocaine addiction will continue to be a serious problem threatens Colombia's future. The continuing civil war and the struggle with the cocaine drug lords have left Colombians exhausted and with little hope. They have a right to be dispirited; although cocaine use in the United States has dropped, it has not reduced the drug business in Colombia. The sale of high quality heroin from Colombia has increased. The Colombian drug cartels have been diversifying since the late 1980s, moving into opium cultivation and heroin production. Consequently, world opium production grew rapidly in the 1990s. The Central Intelligence Agency estimates that opium production increased from 2,000 metric tons in the 1980s to 4,000 metric tons by the mid-1990s. It takes ten tons of raw opium to yield one ton of heroin. Most of the opium is produced in Southeast Asia's Golden Triangle, but Colombia went from zero production of opium to sixty-five metric tons in 1995.

While the major increase in people addicted to heroin was greater in Colombia, where the heroin was produced, toward the end of the twentieth century, the United States and Western Europe were hit with an aggressive heroin marketing campaign led by Nigerian, Chinese, Colombian, and Mexican drug-trafficking rings. The United States has roughly 600,000 heroin addicts or about 2 percent of the world's total heroin addicts (Agence France Presse, 1996). U.S. addicts consume between 10 and 12 tons of heroin a year, or about 3 percent of the heroin that could be produced in a typical year from the worldwide opium poppy crop (McCaffrey, 1996). The remainder of the opium and heroin is consumed by people in the producing and transporting countries. Regardless, the money made from the high-end retail market, the U.S. and Western European market, adds up to enormous profits for those directly and indirectly involved in the illegal drug trade.

Proposed Solutions and Strategies

The increased number of addicts in Colombia is not the result of an increase in weak individuals. Nor can it be dealt with as an individual problem. The illegal drug trade is a corrosive force that fosters corruption, undermines the social order, defies the rule of law, and encourages addiction in every country it touches. In this regard, the illegal drug trade (not the drugs per se) has placed some of the world's most at-risk countries like Colombia in great jeopardy.

In the short term, the only hope for reducing drug production and drug addiction among the people of Colombia is the ongoing Colombian peace process. To move this process forward, human rights violations against the rural peasants and the urban poor by the Colombian government must be stopped. This will give the poor (those most adversely affected by illegal drugs) a chance to reconnect with the government, which, in turn, will reduce the influence of revolutionary groups.

There also must be a change of focus in the war on drugs as directed from Washington. Large-scale crop-substitution programs must be developed in Colombia, as in Bolivia and Peru, and eradication programs reduced. Crop-substitution programs should provide the small Colombian farmer with an income that is competitive with the income they could earn from drug-plant cultivation. This would give rural peasants an alternative to cultivating coca and poppy. Subsequently, this would reduce the raw material available to drug producers.

CONCLUSION

Reducing drug addiction in Colombia is dependent on reducing the cultivation and production of coca and opium in Colombia. This would go a long way toward reducing violence and rebuilding the country's infrastructure and sense of national pride. Nonetheless, if demand for these illegal drugs is not reduced in the United States and Western Europe, driving the drug cartels out of Colombia will not do the rest of the world any good. As the drug traffickers have done before, they will move to another at-risk country and proceed to use it as their illegal drug haven. Destroying the drug traffickers in Colombia would be good for Colombia, but internationally the illegal drug agglomeration would not change.

Treatment for individuals who become addicted is available in Colombia, but it cannot meet the need. Drug-treatment programs vary, but they have a Colombian flavor as a result of adapting U.S. and European treatment models to fit the Colombian culture. In the Colombian model, clinicians reject the medical model of treatment and view addiction as a social problem. They also reject abstinence as a necessary condition for treatment. The Colombian government has little interest, however, in addiction treatment. Given the plethora of other national and social problems, addiction treatment has a low national priority. This can only coalesce to increase the number of people addicted to drugs in Colombia.

A Failed Developmental Policy

The international drug trade did not emerge fully developed from a vacuum. It developed over the years in response to a failed national and international policy intended to help developing countries increase their production of legal and marketable goods. In part, people in source countries such as Colombia, Bolivia, and Peru became involved in the narcotic business after the widespread international and national failure in these countries to develop legitimate routes to economic prosperity and growth for the people of the Andean region of South America.

REFERENCES

Agence France Presse. (1996, November 28). *Opium production increasing dramatically—report.* Paris, France: Author.

Brecher, E.M. (1972). *Licit and illicit drugs.* Boston: Little Brown.

Bushnell, D. (1993). *The making of modern Colombia: A nation in spite of itself.* Los Angeles: University of California Press.

Encarta Desk Encyclopedia. (1998). *Colombia.* Microsoft Corporation [CD-ROM].

Hall, K.G. (2000, October 18). Colombia plan won't be a Vietnam, Cohen vows. *Miami Herald,* p. 5A.

Hanratty, D.M., and Meditz, S.W. (1988). *Colombia—A country study.* Washington, DC: Federal Research Division, Library of Congress.

Ivins, M. (1999, November 5). US should help stop Columbian madness. *Los Angeles Times,* p. 30. Downloaded from the World Wide Web, September 9, 2000, http://www.amazoncoalition.org

The Latin America Working Group. (1999). *Act now! Just say no to Colombia military aid.* Washington, DC: Author.

Marquez, G.G. (1997). *Goodfella: News of a kidnapping.* New York: Alfred A. Knopf.

McCaffrey, B. (1996, September 19). *Heroin : A global threat.* Washington, DC: Federal News Service.

Ministerio de Salud. (1996). *Boletin epidemiologico nacional* (National epidemiological bulletin). Bogotá: Author.

Monastero, F. (1985). *Consultant paper: Recommendations for the regulation of selected chemicals and controlled substance analogs.* Washington, DC: Drug Enforcement Administration.

Montoya, I.D., & Chilcoat, H.D. (1996). Epidemiology of coca derivatives use in the Andean region: A tale of five countries. *Substance Use and Misuse, 31,* 1227–1240.

Pérez-Gómez, A. (1998). Drug consumption and drug treatment in a drug-producing country: Columbia between myth and reality—A view from inside. In H. Klingemann & G. Hunt (Eds.), *Drug treatment systems in an international perspective: Drugs, demons, and delinquents* (pp. 173–181). Thousand Oaks, CA: Sage Publications.

Rosenberg, C. (2001, April 26). CIA Grounds Missions in Colombia and Peru. *Miami Herald,* p. 1A.

Schemo, D.J. (1998a, February 28). Colombian peasants seek way out of drug trade. *New York Times,* sec. A, p. 1

———. (1998b, March 2). Colombia farmers stuck with drugs; funds to switch crops unavailable. *International Herald Tribune* (France), p. 3.

Toxic war. (2000, July 13). *Boston Globe,* p. A20.

U.S. Senate. (1994, March). *Money laundering—U.s. efforts to fight it are threatened by currency smuggling*. Submitted to the Chairman, Permanent Subcommittee on Investigations, Committee on Governmental Affairs U.S. Senate. GAO/GGD-94-73.

Zeese, K.B. (2000, March 29). Ignoring lessons of drug wars past. *The Progressive Response*, 4 (13), 3–29.

5

ENGLAND

Douglas Rugh

INTRODUCTION

England was once considered progressive in dealing with its drug and alcohol problem. Other countries spent a great deal of time studying the English approaches to heroin and alcohol treatment. Recently, however, the United Kingdom's drug policy has changed its focus from providing treatment for individual drug dependents to protecting the community. As a part of the ten-year drug strategy, the new Labor government has appointed a drug czar, which moved England from a harm-reduction model more to a prohibition model. A major thrust of the new strategy is to reduce drug-related crime. It is estimated that 3 percent of the 4 million people who use illicit drugs each year have serious drug problems; of these, between 100,000 and 200,000 may each spend an average of £200 (U.S.$280) per week to fund their habits. Approximately 20 percent of those passing through the criminal justice system have a drug problem and would benefit from treatment (Martin, 1999). Often health problems, poverty, developmental problems, and crimes are associated with untreated drug use. This chapter examines this problem and explores Britain's options for the immediate future.

A Brief Profile of England

The population of England in 2000 was estimated to be more than 59 million people. The population density was about 1,100 people per square mile, or about 430 people per square kilometer. The United Kingdom is a country with one of the highest population densities in the world. Seventy-five percent of the people live in urban areas; only 25 percent of the land can be cultivated (*Encarta Desk Encyclopedia*, 1998).

Most English people are descended from early Celtic, Iberian peoples and from Nordic and French invaders. In the year 2000, the United Kingdom comprised England, and regional assemblies with varying degrees of power in Scotland, Wales, and Northern Ireland. The country of England occupies the entire island east of Wales and south of Scotland. The chief port is London. Its total area is 50,363 square miles (130, 439 square kilometers), including the Isles of Scilly, the Isle of Wight, and the Isle of Man (*Encarta Desk Encyclopedia*, 1998).

The gross domestic product (GDP) per capita in England (a measure of individual buying power) was estimated in 1999 to be $21,800 (in U.S. currency) per person per year. An estimated 17 percent of the people have incomes below the poverty line. Unemployment is typically about 6 percent.

Life expectancy at birth in England is consistent with the best of the developed nations. For the total population it is slightly more than 77.5 years. For males, it is just under 75 years and for females, it is an impressive 80.5 years. Using a definition of literacy that includes all English citizens age fifteen and over who have completed five or more years of schooling, the literacy rate in the United Kingdom is 99 percent for the total population (*Encarta Desk Encyclopedia*, 1998). School attendance is compulsory from ages six through sixteen, and elementary and secondary schools are primarily organized and maintained by public funds. The oldest of England's many institutions of higher education are the universities of Oxford and Cambridge.

English law originated in the customs of the Anglo-Saxons and the Normans. England's basic legal documents, including the Magna Carta and the Bill of Rights, with their emphasis on the legal rights of the individual, have influenced the entire English-speaking world (*Encarta Desk Encyclopedia*, 1998). The Church of England, a Protestant Episcopalian denomination, is the state church and the church of nearly 60 percent of the population. Catholics, other Protestant denominations, Muslims, and Jews make up the remainder.

England is a constitutional monarchy consisting of a sovereign ruler, the House of Commons, and the House of Lords. In modern times, the monarchy and the House of Lords have been ceremonial institutions with little or no real authority. Under the central government, the nation is divided into 30 nonmetropolitan counties, six metropolitan counties, and Greater London (established in 1965 as a separate administrative entity) (*Encarta Desk Encyclopedia*, 1998).

VIGNETTE

The following vignette is a fictional interview between a reporter and a medical researcher. The reporter is interviewing the scientist about England's use of medical clinics to distribute heroin to the country's registered addicts.

Scientist: The choices we have are drugs from the clinic or drugs from the Mafia. A gram of 100 percent pure heroin on the streets would be cut 10 to 15 times and £1,390 ($2,000). Take it away from the black market, make it legal, and heroin is a cheap drug. The British National Health Service (NHS) pays about £6.93 ($10.00) for a gram of heroin.

Reporter: To get drugs from the clinic rather than the Mafia, addicts submit a urine test to prove they are taking the drug they say they are. And unlike most other addiction clinics where you have to say you want to kick the habit before they'll take you in, addicts here intend to stay on drugs. But can clinics try to cure people?

Scientist: Cure people? Nobody can. Regardless of whether you stick them in prison, put them in mental hospitals and give them shock treatment, we have done all these things, put them in a nice rehab center away in the country, give them a nice social worker and pat them on the head, give them drugs, give them no drugs—does not matter what you do. Five percent per annum, 1 in 20 per year, get off spontaneously. Compounded, that means about 50 percent are off drugs after 10 years. People seem to mature out of addiction regardless of any intervention. In the interim, we can keep them alive, healthy, and legal during those ten years.

Reporter: By giving them drugs?

Scientist: Narcotics do not get them off drugs; it doesn't prolong their addiction, either. But it stops them from breaking the law, it keeps them healthy and it keeps them alive.

Reporter: That's exactly what happened to Wendy. She is a heroin addict. For the last three years, the heroin she injects every day comes from a prescription. Before, she fed her habit by working as a prostitute. A harmful cycle that led to sexually transmitted diseases, hepatitis, and more heroin to cope with her lifestyle. Once they have gotten their prescriptions, addicts must participate in regular meetings to show that they are staying healthy and free from crime.

Scientist: Pure heroin is not dangerous. We have people on massive doses of heroin. The street heroin that is causing damage is not because of the heroin; it is because of the bread dust, coffee, or crushed bleach crystals. Heroin can be 90 percent adulterated with harmful chemicals. If you inject glue into your veins, you don't have to be a medical expert to know that you are causing harm.

Reporter: In the 1970s the British were not content with minimizing the harm of drug abuse. They adopted the American policy of trying to stop it all together. Prescriptions were no longer widely available. Addicts who couldn't kick the habit had to find illegal sources. By the end of the 1980s drug addiction in Britain had tripled.

Reporter: Tom is one who has settled into a regular, sensible life on cocaine. He has a prescription for both cocaine spray and cocaine cigarettes. Before he got that prescription, the cocaine he bought on the street cost him nearly $1,000 a week, which at first he managed to take from his own business, but it wasn't long before it cost him much more than that. He lost his business, he lost his wife, he lost his kids and the house, but he kept going after the cocaine. Now, after two years of controlled use, Tom has voluntarily reduced his dose, and he has a regular job.

Scientist: The whole concept behind that is control. There are signs that control is working. Within the area of the clinic, the police have reported a significant drop in drug related crime and since addicts don't have to deal anymore to support their habit, they're not recruiting new customers. So, far fewer new people are being turned on to drugs.

OVERVIEW OF SOCIAL ISSUE AND BASIC DEMOGRAPHICS

Marijuana is the most popular prohibited drug in the United Kingdom. However, with more than 100,000 heroin addicts, a major concern of British officials is stemming the abuse of heroin and other injected drugs. There has been an increase in crack cocaine and cocaine use. British authorities are concerned about the use of amphetamines and Ecstasy, particularly among young people. Methadone is also frequently misused.

Marijuana is cultivated in limited amounts in the United Kingdom for personal use using hydroponic growing systems, and it occasionally is sold for commercial use. When such cultivation is detected, authorities destroy the crops and facilities. Amphetamines and Ecstasy are also manufactured in limited amounts in clandestine laboratories which are destroyed by the authorities when found.

Steady supplies of heroin and cocaine enter the United Kingdom. The bulk of heroin originates in the Golden Crescent of Southwest Asia, notably in Afghanistan and Pakistan, and is routed through Iran, Turkey (where much of it is processed), and Central Europe. Marijuana comes primarily from Morocco. Large cocaine shipments arrive directly from South America; smaller shipments often come up from the Spanish coast, either directly to the United Kingdom or via Amsterdam. There is also a synthetic drug market that originates out of Western and Central Europe. Amphetamines, Ecstasy, and LSD have been traced from clandestine laboratories in the Netherlands and Poland, as well as in the United Kingdom.

The Cost of Addiction

Alcohol is part of the European cultural tradition, with a significant recreational role. Consumed in small quantities, it can have health benefits for certain groups. But alcohol is also an addictive drug and a major cause of ill health and social distress. It plays a role in liver cirrhosis, cancers, and heart disease, and its misuse places families under stress, causes unemployment and homelessness, and affects the wider community in terms of violence, disorder, and accidents.

While economic benefits are associated with the alcohol industry, the financial costs to society of alcohol misuse are substantial. They involve health, welfare, and criminal justice services' costs, as well as the financial implications of unemployment and lost productivity. One calculation suggests an overall figure of £10 billion (U.S.$14 billion) per year (Alcohol Concern, 1999).

A report published by Alcohol Concern (AC) states that "one person in 20 is dependent on alcohol—compared with one in 45, who is hooked on any other form of legal or illegal drug, including prescription drugs." AC outlined the major areas they wanted the government to address in their National Alcohol Strategy in May 1999. These areas included taxation, licensing laws and hours, advertising and packaging, as well as campaigns to promote care with alcohol. The report also found that young people were drinking regularly, with children between the ages of eleven and fifteen years old consuming, on an average, twice as much as they did in 1990. In addition, £2.8 billion (U.S.$3 billion) sterling is being lost by British industry each year from alcohol-related absence, unemployment, and premature death. Alcohol abuse is also linked with 65 percent of the suicide attempts made annually (Alcohol Concern, 1999).

HISTORY OF ALCOHOL AND DRUG USE IN ENGLAND

Physicians in the United Kingdom are permitted by law to prescribe any drug except opium for their patients. This practice dates back to a committee put together by Sir Humphrey Rolleston during the 1920s. The Rolleston Committee was a group of leading physicians experienced in the treatment of dependent drug users. One of the most significant conclusions of the committee was the following:

When . . . every effort possible in the circumstances has been made, and made unsuccessfully, to bring the patient to a condition in which he is independent of the drug, it may . . . become justifiable in certain cases to order regularly the minimum dose which has been found necessary, either in order to avoid serious withdrawal symptoms, or to keep the patient in a condition in which he can lead a useful life. (Riley, 1998)

Although there have been some important changes to the British system in response to the changing nature of the user population and tightening of controls over physicians, in many ways the recommendations of the Rolleston report are still being followed. This is particularly true in the Mersey region in northwestern England where services follow the philosophy that even if you can not "cure" dependence, you can still care for drug users by providing injectable opiates and other drugs to registered users. The local police ensure the success of this approach by not placing drug services under observation and by referring drug users to these services. The majority of clients receive oral methadone, but some receive injectable methadone, others injectable heroin, and a small number amphetamines, cocaine, or other drugs. These drugs are dispensed through local pharmacists. In some parts of the United Kingdom, users can also be prescribed smokable drugs.

SUBSTANCE ABUSE IN ENGLAND TODAY

Political Views and Public Policies

British drug policy addresses demand reduction, treatment, and law enforcement, and focuses on locally based action plans. The United Kingdom has developed a ten-year strategy, outlined in a white paper issued in April 1998, entitled *Tackling Drugs to Build a Better Britain*. This strategy builds upon old ones, but it puts greater stress on the importance of all sectors of society working together to combat drugs. Its new focus recognizes that drug problems do not occur in isolation and are often linked to other social problems. The strategy is a part of a wider UK government program for tackling reforms in the welfare state, education, employment, health, criminal justice, and the economy. The strategy has four elements:

1. To help young people resist drug misuse, in order to achieve their full potential in society;
2. To protect communities from drug-related, antisocial and criminal behavior;
3. To enable people with drug problems to overcome them and live healthy, crime-free lives; and,
4. To stifle the availability of drugs on the streets.

The new strategy has been accompanied by a wide-scale review of the resources available for tackling drug misuse. The government spends around U.S.$2.3 billion a year tackling the problem—62 percent (U.S.$1.43 billion) of this total goes to enforcement-related work. The other, 38 percent (U.S.$870 million) is spent on education, prevention, and treatment. The new strategy marks a progressive shift away from reactive expenditure, like dealing with the consequences of drug misuse, toward a greater investment in prevention.

In September 1998, the government announced an additional $358 million over the next three years for antidrug projects. This includes $99 million for the new drug treatment and testing order and $123 million toward a comprehensive provision for the treatment of problem drug abusers in prison and their rehabilitation back into society. In addition, $115 million is available for setting up new community-based treatment services.

The United Kingdom vigorously contributes to international drug-control efforts. With the new drug strategy in mind, this assistance has focused on the Southwest Asia and Balkan heroin route, as well as the Latin America and Caribbean cocaine route. The country strongly supports and works closely with the United Nations Drugs Control Program (UNDCP). The British play a leading role in a number of international drug-control forums including the Council of Europe's Pompidou Group, the Dublin Group, EUROPOL's Drug Unit and other EU forums, and the Financial Action Task Force (FATF). The United Kingdom chairs the southwest drug unit in the Dublin Group and is an active counter-narcotics advocate in the many mini-Dublin groups throughout the world.

The drug treatment and testing order is a new community sentence, which enables courts to require drug offenders to undergo treatment and to submit to mandatory and random drug testing to ensure that they remain clean. The new order was put into effect in three areas of England in September 30, 1998. New legislation to enable nightclubs and similar venues to be closed immediately when found to harbor a serious drug problem was brought into effect on May 1, 1998. This new enforcement power has been little used to date, but it appears to have helped considerably in encouraging club operators to improve security and increase vigilance against drug misuse.

British law enforcement officials, including customs and excise officials, are vigilant and effective. In November 1998, Home Office Secretary Jack Straw put forward for public consultation ways in which the United Kingdom can improve upon the seizure of assets from criminals, primarily drug dealers. Procedures for civil asset forfeiture were proposed in a white paper policy document.

The government's demand reduction efforts focus on school and other community-based programs to educate young people and prevent them from taking drugs. Additionally, the Drug Prevention Advisory Service reestablished school and community teams involved in this activity from April 1999. These teams will give specialist prevention advice to all of the locally based drug-action teams.

Since 1989 the governments of the United States and the United Kingdom have conducted periodic consultations at the senior level to coordinate and harmonize policies, plans, and programs on all counter-narcotics fronts. Law enforcement cooperation between the two countries is excellent and growing. The United Kingdom cooperates with efforts made by the United States and other countries to trace or seize illicit assets. British laws permit the sharing of forfeited assets with the United States. Asset sharing with other nations is both formal and ad hoc.

Social Views, Customs, and Practices

The Mersey region has the second highest rate of notified addicts of any regional health authority in the United Kingdom; however, the level of HIV infection among drug injectors in the Mersey region is very low, less than 1 percent. There have been significant decreases in crime related to property, robbery of pharmacies, and break-and-enters. Since no experimental trials or controlled studies have been conducted in this region, the data are considered to be too unreliable for the purposes of setting policy in other countries. The Mersey model has been followed successfully in most parts of the United Kingdom, with a national average of only 1 percent HIV infection in injection drug users. The police policy of "cautioning" for small amounts for personal use has now been extended to all drugs and is practiced throughout the country (Riley, 1998).

There has been a significant increase in the numbers of women and young adult men drinking above sensible limits, as well as a rise in the frequency of drinking and the amount of alcohol consumed by children.

THE FUTURE OF SUBSTANCE ABUSE IN ENGLAND

The government's statutory Advisory Council on the Misuse of Drugs (ACMD) stated in 1988 that AIDS was a greater threat to public health than drug misuse, and it recommended that drug services modify their policies to make contact with and change the behavior of the maximum number of drug users even when they are still actively using drugs. The ACMD advised that drug services proceed according to the hierarchy of objectives for behavior change, starting with the cessation of sharing injection equipment followed by a switch to non-injecting drug use, a reduction in drug use, and, ultimately, cessation of drug use.

Increased medical understanding of the effects of alcohol consumption have led to an awareness that the health risks do not apply only to heavier dependent drinkers, but also to those who drink somewhat in excess of sensible limits—some 20 percent of the adult population. There is also a greater recognition of the spectrum of social harms caused by alcohol misuse and their impact on a community's safety and quality of life.

Proposed Solutions and Strategies

A strategic approach is required to ensure that action is taken to tackle these problems, and to provide a framework for resolving the wide range of complementary and divergent commercial, recreational, and welfare interests associated with alcohol consumption. To meet concerns over the fragmented nature of alcohol policy development, there is a need to coordinate the large number of agencies with a stake in alcohol policy, including at least ten government departments, and to ensure that alcohol issues are addressed within the context of new government multisectored initiatives in related fields.

Although the debate continues in political circles and among professional human service providers, it has moved from campaigns to stop addiction to programs that punish addicts. Politicians and the public will realize that the drug problem will not disappear simply because the person has been locked in jail for a few years.

CONCLUSION

There is no country in the world that has reached 100 percent prohibition of illegal drugs. England's attempts at treating the problem were having a positive effect on the population, although drugs and alcohol remained a continuing problem. It appears that instead of decreasing society's acceptance levels, it would be wiser to increase our levels of tolerance. Drugs and alcohol are a part of our world, and the more we try to eradicate them from society the more problems we create. By focusing on the human element and vigorously attempting to change behavior, England can return to a higher threshold of tolerance, which eventually will stabilize drug and alcohol abuse among its population.

REFERENCES

Alcohol Concern. (1999). Proposals for a national alcohol strategy for England. London.

Bureau for International Narcotics and Law Enforcement Affairs (1999, March). *International Narcotics Control Strategy Report*. Washington, D.C. Downloaded on November 11, 2000, from www.usis.usemb.se/drugs/1998.

Encarta Desk Encyclopedia (1998). Microsoft Corporation [CD-ROM].

Martin, P. (1999, April). Abstract for international symposium on substance abuse treatment and special target groups, "Managing Change." De Haan, Belgium.

Riley, D. (1998). *Drug and drug policy in Canada: A brief review and commentary*. Ottawa: Canadian Foundation for Drug Policy.

6

FRANCE

Andrew Cherry and Louis B. Antoine

INTRODUCTION

Although some may argue about which wine is the best from year to year, the majority of wine connoisseurs agree that France is the premier wine-producing country in the world. French wine comes from grapes grown on small French farms, usually less than 40 hectares (100 acres). The wines from these vineyards are considered to be among the highest-quality wines in the world. For centuries, the French have taken their wine very seriously. It is a source of national pride. The French classify their wines by the region of France in which the grapes are grown. The most famous are the Bordeaux region, located along the southwestern coast; and the Burgundy region, located in central France. In the 1990s French wine production reached about 6.2 billion liters (approximately 1.6 billion gallons) a year. Not surprisingly, France leads the world in the production of wine (Buck, 1997).

Tax on French Wine

The tax on French wine is very low because it is not meant to generate revenue for the state, or to act as a deterrent to the production or consumption of French wine in France. The tax on French wine is only intended to provide the French government with the financing needed to monitor the production, distribution, and consumption of French wine. The purpose of the monitoring is to ensure that French wines sold under the name of a specific wine-growing region of France are authentic. This helps maintain the worldwide reputation of French wine and increases its commercial value (Buck, 1997).

Alcoholism in France

The French tradition of drinking wine at almost every occasion and with every meal has resulted in an ethnically related drug problem—an estimated 5 million French people are at risk of medical, psychological, and social problems; and 2 million more people are dependent on alcohol in France. The consumption of alcohol, usually in the form of wine, has actually declined in France. In 1970 the French yearly consumed 22 liters (about 5 gallons) of unadulterated alcohol for every man, woman, and child in France. In the form of wine, this amount of alcohol is close to 170 liters (180 quarts) of wine per person per year, or slightly over a pint of wine a day. In 1989 consumption had dropped to 17 liters (18 quarts) per person per year. The drop in consumption came as good news because it typically indicates a corresponding drop in alcohol-related problems. In France, this is important. Even after the drop in alcohol consumption, a 1991 survey found that about 1,000 cases of fetal alcohol syndrome births were still occurring each year. Also, between 15 and 35 percent of emergency service and hospital beds were taken up by victims of alcohol abuse, primarily psychiatric hospital beds. The study also found that 29.5 percent of French men and 11.1 percent of French women seen by general practitioners were seen because of excessive drinking (more than twenty-eight drinks per week for men and fourteen drinks per week for women). At this level of alcohol consumption over an extended period of time, a person is at risk of alcohol-related disease or is already ill (Institute of Alcohol Studies, 1997).

Excessive alcohol consumption is responsible for many health problems in France (damage to the peripheral and central nervous systems, liver, cardiovascular system, and an unborn child). It is also a determining factor in many social problems, ranging from job problems to criminal behavior (violent attacks, rape, child abuse, and domestic abuse). In some circumstances, such as driving, alcohol consumption considerably increases the risk of accidents.

Male life expectancy in France has been affected by the heavy consumption of alcohol. The male life expectancy in France is 72.9 years compared with Japan (75.9), Sweden (74.9), Italy (74.0), Spain (73.3), and the United Kingdom (73.2). Most of this difference is due to accidents, alcohol, and smoking. The mortality rate in France (compared with Great Britain, West Germany, Italy, and the Netherlands) is very high among boys and young men. Accidents (51 percent) and suicide (12.5 percent) are the two main factors. People between eighteen and twenty-four years of age represent 10.5 percent of the French population, but they account for 25 percent of the accidental deaths. Furthermore, in 1991, 800 young people committed suicide, and 40,000 suicide attempts were made by young people under the age of twenty-five ("High Committee Report Sheds New Light," 1997).

The Drug Problem in France

In addition to the problem of alcohol addiction, the French have a serious problem with illegal drug use and addiction. Although it started to level off and even drop in the late 1990s, it is still a serious concern for health officials. In 1997 heroin seizures dropped 32.7 percent, and there was a decrease of 18.7 percent in the number of people arrested for selling and using heroin. This would suggest that the actual use of heroin had also dropped. This drop in heroin use for two years in a row was the first major drop in more than twenty years of increased heroin use. French officials noted, however, that heroin had always been used by a small proportion of the French people. Cannabis and Ecstasy, they point out, continue to be the most widely abused drugs in France at the beginning of the twenty-first century. Although the number of French heroin users began to drop toward the end of the 1990s, heroin and drug trafficking in general continued to be a concern to French law enforcement officials (U.S. Department of State, 1999).

Cocaine consumption began to increase in the 1990s and had spread into the middle economic classes by the mid-1990s. Cannabis (primarily hashish) consumption continues to be viewed as a serious problem, particularly among teens between fourteen and eighteen years of age. Another major drug concern among French officials at the beginning of the twenty-first century was an increase in the use of Ecstasy by persons ranging in age from sixteen to thirty.

Like other European countries, France is increasingly facing the problem of polydrug addiction. Moreover, drug addiction will likely continue to be a problem in France for some time to come because of France's role as a drug transit country, the same role it played in the movie *The French Connection*. Although very little heroin is smuggled into the United States from France (as it was when the French connection was in operation), France now supplies other European countries with illegal drugs. They wholesale heroin from Turkey and Southwest Asia, cocaine from South America, hashish (cannabis) from Morocco, and Ecstasy from the Netherlands (Korf and Riper, 1977). To deal effectively with the drug problem in France, prohibition policies are slowly being changed by French officials who are cautiously adopting a public health model similar to the model used by other EU countries.

A Brief Profile of France

The population of France is estimated to be at about 59 million people. The labor force numbers over 25 million men and women. In 1998 the

GDP was close to $1.32 trillion. France has managed to maintain an inflation rate below 1 percent and is firmly established among the premier industrialized nations of the world. The per capita income is $22,600. France spends a significant percentage of its resources on its health care system. With the government overseeing the location of hospitals and maintaining a strict bed/population ratio, the French citizenry is free to choose treatment in a number of private or public hospitals. There is one physician for every 334 patients and one hospital per 15,000 people. In 1998 the average amount of money reimbursed by social security per person for health care was 12,270 francs (U.S.$2,250) per person. The percentage of GNP spent on health care in France remains well below that of the United States—9.8 percent in France and 14.2 percent in the United States (Central Intelligence Agency, 2000).

The life expectancy in France is 72.9 years for males and 82.7 years for females, a large and expanding geriatric group (20 percent of the population is over sixty). There were 11.38 live births per 1,000 population and 9.17 deaths per 1,000 in 1999. Some 26 percent of the general population remains under twenty years of age. The infant mortality rate is among the lowest in the world at 5.62 deaths per 1,000 live births (Central Intelligence Agency, 2000).

Although France has a relatively high unemployment rate by industrialized nation standards (11.5 percent in 1998), very few French people live below the poverty level. On the recent United Nations Human Development Report which surveyed 174 nations (measuring personal income, access to health care, education, and life expectancy), France ranked twelfth behind such countries as Canada, Norway, the United States, and Finland.

In France, the predominant ethnic groups are Celtic and Latin with some Teutonic, Slavic, and North African in the minority. The population is 90 percent Roman Catholic, 2 percent Protestant, 1 percent Jewish, and 1 percent Muslim; 6 percent claim no religious affiliation. Education is readily available to all, and the literacy rate, which is defined as the percentage of the population of fifteen-year-olds and over that can read and write, is 99 percent (*Encarta Desk Encyclopedia*, 1998).

VIGNETTE

In May 1970, President Richard Nixon sent a new ambassador to France, Arthur Watson, the former chairman of International Business Machines (IBM). Watson's instructions from Nixon were simple: "Your job is to clean up the heroin problem in France. That is the most important priority today." When Watson arrived in Paris (with his copy of the book *The French Connection*), he was surprised to discover that the French had no interest in heroin addiction or the heroin problem. The French considered it an "American disease." The Central Intelligence Agency (CIA) estimated that the vast majority of heroin that was smuggled into the United States went through Marseilles. This was also where labs converted the morphine base into heroin.

Ambassador Watson, being from the world of U.S. business, knew that the only way to get French officials to act against the heroin producers and traffickers was to convince the French people that heroin was also a French problem. To this end, Watson's operatives planted stories in French newspapers about heroin addicts in France, and to no one's surprise, the public-relations campaign worked. The French people's concern about heroin went from zero in the French polls to the number one problem. Moreover, the press campaign led to a doubling of drug-enforcement policies in France, and French officials became more cooperative. Nevertheless, this did not satisfy the Nixon administration. Telegrams from the State Department and the White House kept asking when a "major heroin lab in Marseilles would be seized." After several investigations, Watson realized that the infamous heroin-making labs were "no more than dirty kitchens" where trays of morphine base were cooked with acetic anhydride until the base became heroin. To Watson's dismay, any house in Marseilles, or for that matter any house in the world with running water, could be converted to a heroin lab. Agents with the French Bureau of Narcotics were also skeptical about the value of seizing heroin labs because such operations could be moved from one kitchen to another in a few days. As far as the Nixon administration was concerned, this was an excuse. The president, congressional representatives, and American journalists wanted the French to bust a few heroin labs. And, being used to success at IBM, the ambassador was determined to seize as many dirty kitchens as he could, with or without French help or approval.

His first step was to assign the embassy's science attaché full time to the problem of finding heroin labs. Next, the ambassador, piloting his own propjet plane, flew to Marseilles, where he and the attaché met with French police in the same restaurant that was used in the opening scene of the movie *The French Connection*. There they discussed the operations of the heroin labs: import, manufacture, and trafficking. After several meetings, they came up with the idea of "sniffing out" the acetic anhydrides used in heroin production. The company that developed a technique in Vietnam to determine the presence of drugs in urine was given the contract to develop a heroin "sniffer." In 1971 the sniffer was ready to be tested. Concealed in a Volkswagen bus with a snorkel-like pipe protruding out the roof, American agents drove through the streets of Marseilles sniffing out heroin drug labs, charting the signals indicating acetic anhydrides on a street map. Although they were able to identify many sites, they found, to their dismay, that acetic acid is indistinguishable from the strong odor of vinaigrette salad dressing. When the sites on the map were checked, they found they had inadvertently identified a number of good restaurants, but no heroin labs. To the great amusement of the French officials, the sniffer was sent back to the United States.

Ambassador Watson's next idea was to go into the sewers of Marseilles.

He observed that the water used in the production of heroin would contain telltale traces of the materials needed to make heroin. By sampling the sewage and following the water, one could identify the heroin labs. Because the ambassador had no budget, he invited a "secret and unorthodox group" (the CIA) to run the operation. For the next few months, American agents waded in the sewers of Marseilles collecting sewer water from different areas of the city to no avail. No heroin labs could be found.

Although the sewer escapade did not result in finding any heroin labs, it did convince French officials of the resolve of the Americans. They realized that the Americans would never give up on the idea of seizing some of the heroin drug labs in Marseilles. Therefore, to placate the ambassador and the Nixon administration, the French police moved in. They rounded up their local informants and the few drug addicts they knew and, with the information from these sources, they raided about a half dozen heroin lab kitchens, thus appeasing Nixon, a large number of congressmen, and American journalists (Epstein, 1977). This action may actually have contributed to a heroin problem in France—if heroin was too costly to ship to the United States, the traffickers reasoned, more of it could be sold locally.

OVERVIEW OF SUBSTANCE ABUSE IN FRANCE AND BASIC DEMOGRAPHICS

The French have one drug in common: the alcohol in the wine they produce and drink or the alcohol from cheap Algerian wine, depending on what one can afford. The young also have their own drug in common: marijuana. The role played by marijuana or hashish in sporadic youth rebellions convinced many in France that cannabis was a part of the larger youth problem. Consequently, for years the French have been debating their policy on cannabis use. The debate, until recently, was over the definition of zero tolerance and cannabis use, and arguments about law enforcement's not being strict enough on cannabis users. In the 1990s, however, there was a shift in the debate. Advocates for a less harmful drug policy called attention to the effect of decriminalization of cannabis use in other EU countries, particularly England, Germany, and Holland (Chabrol, Callahan, and Fredaigue, 2000).

In 1994 a number of prestigious French committees and organizations came out in favor of the decriminalization of cannabis use. Although the government was not willing to follow those recommendations, the growing consensus in France, and in the world, was that people who use cannabis should not be jailed or punished simply for using cannabis.

Cannabis in France for the most part means Moroccan hash. Over 80 percent of the cannabis on the French illegal drug market is in the form of hashish from Morocco. Although hash from other countries, such as Afghanistan and Pakistan, can be found, there is not much of it. Marijuana is even more difficult to find. The marijuana that is sold comes from the Caribbean, Africa, or the Netherlands. There are a few marijuana farmers in the south of France, but these are small-scale growers who sell the crop to friends and established consumers (Chabrol, Callahan, and Fredaigue, 2000).

Traffickers in hashish, in France, are typically small-scale operators living in the *banlieues*, the working-class suburbs. These communities are characterized by inexpensive high-rise apartments, unemployment, and a high proportion of immigrants, especially people from North Africa (Algeria, Morocco, and Tunisia). Drug trafficking in these communities is often looked upon as a way out of poverty and dead-end jobs, which makes for a thriving underground, illegal drug economy that flourishes in these French suburban communities (Buck, 1997).

The Prevalence of Cannabis Use in France

Roughly 4.7 million French people between the ages of twelve and forty-four have at one time or another smoked cannabis. This represents a lifetime prevalence of 19 percent of all French people. According to a number of studies that have been conducted by the French Committee of Health Education, between 30 and 40 percent of the people between eighteen and thirty-four have at one time or another used cannabis. In another study, the French National Institute of Health and Medical Research found the prevalence of cannabis use at secondary schools to be 12 percent among adolescents between eleven and nineteen years of age, but higher among older teens. Twenty-nine percent of eighteen- or nineteen-year-olds had smoked cannabis at least once. Among those who had ever used cannabis, 40 percent belonged to the regular users group: those who had used cannabis at least ten times in their lives (Boekhout van Solinge, 1997).

HISTORY OF ALCOHOL AND DRUG USE IN FRANCE

The debate over the harm caused by cannabis has a long history in France. The French poet Charles Baudelaire (1821–1867) may have started the debate when he said, "*S'il existait un gouvernement qui eût intérêt à corrompre ses gouvernés, il n'aurait qu'à encourager l'usage du cannabis*" (If there were a government who had interest in corrupting its citizens, it only had to encourage the use of cannabis). Starting from this philosophical position, the aim of the French drug policy was to prevent cannabis use. Accordingly, although the law is not as strictly enforced as it was, the punishment can still be quite severe.

Before 1970 people who used drugs in private were not to be prosecuted. However, after the youth protests in 1968, the drug laws of the 1970s were enforced, especially against young cannabis users. A new drug law in 1994 differentiated between drug possession and drug use. The penalties for cannabis use under this law varies from two months to a year and/or a fine of between 500 and 25,000 francs. The more serious crimes, such as possession for sale, cultivation, and trafficking of cannabis, are punished much more severely. Jail terms of up to ten years and a fine of between 500,000 and 50 million French francs are common.

During the 1980s, the Ministry of Justice issued several directives concerning the prosecution of drug users. Some of these directives called for not prosecuting cannabis users. Since federal directives in France are subordinate to the law, the head prosecutors in each of the 180 districts enforced the policy in different ways. Where cannabis use and possession of small amounts of cannabis (for personal use) was not prosecuted in one part of France, in other places the law might be vigorously enforced. In large cities, there was a growing tolerance of cannabis and other drug use by the police, especially in the lower-class areas like the *banlieues*. In the rural areas cannabis users are often prosecuted (Boekhout van Solinge, 1997).

Nothing much changed until 1995 when the Henrion Commission, the official French state commission charged with reconsidering the French drug policy on cannabis, issued its report. Not only was the commission in favor of decriminalizing cannabis, but after a period of gradual introduction, the commission wanted to institutionalize the retail sale of cannabis. The day the Henrion Commission published its report, Prime Minister Edouard Balladur declared on national television that the French drug policy would not be changed.

SUBSTANCE ABUSE IN FRANCE TODAY

If you compare these and other French data on cannabis use, despite years of prohibition, France is still on the high side of cannabis use in the EU. Buying, selling, and possessing cannabis are considered serious criminal offenses, and in most cases the accused person is prosecuted. Although someone caught using cannabis may not be prosecuted, this does not mean cannabis use is tolerated. Someone using cannabis or found to be carrying a small quantity of cannabis, for example, during a police identity control check, is still taken to the police station and booked. While he or she may not be prosecuted, there is a good chance he or she will be taken into custody and will have to spend the night in prison, making him or her late for school or work the next day.

Political Views and Public Policies

France's drug-control agency, La Mission Interministerielle de Lutte contre la Drogue et la Toxicomanie (MILDT), underwent internal changes in the mid-1990s which improved its ability to set and coordinate France's national policy among the many different departments involved in illegal drug control. In addition, MILDT's mandate was expanded to include alcohol and tobacco. Elements of the policy include integrating efforts against the abuse of tobacco, alcohol, and legal drugs. France's antinarcotics programs now focus more on repressing drug trafficking (and particularly local trafficking) than arresting drug users. The policy does not require the authorities to arrest a drug user for "simple usage." In fact, prevention is focused on preventing occasional users from becoming abusers and on preventing abusers from developing an addiction. This policy was based on the seriousness of the illegal behavior of the drug user rather than on the toxicity of the drug used.

Law Enforcement

French counter-narcotics authorities have been quite busy since the late 1970s. In 1998 French authorities in southeastern France arrested thirty members of an organization that smuggled Colombian cocaine into France and other European countries from South America via Venezuela, Guyana, and the Dutch Antilles. An investigation conducted by the Police Judiciaire of Marseille also led to the arrest of nineteen people involved in cocaine trafficking from Colombia via Spain to France. In the spring of 1998, over 3,000 police and customs officers from France, Belgium, the Netherlands, Germany, and Luxembourg participated in an enforcement operation that targeted different drug-trafficking routes. The operation reportedly resulted in significant heroin, hashish, and cocaine seizures. Nevertheless, figures on drug arrests over the same period in France show that approximately 75 percent of those arrested were drug users, but only 10 percent of those arrested were dealers (Mossé, 1998).

Alcohol Tax on Beer and Whisky

Alcoholic beverage taxation is somewhat different in France than in other EU countries. This turned into a controversy when, in the late 1990s, the French government came under attack by both brewers and distillers for their increased taxes on alcohol. In October 1996, the government announced that it would increase the tax on spirits by 17.1 percent. French and British spirit companies sued the French government, saying that the tax was unfair because the tax did not apply to French wine.

Consequently, the EU commission regulating taxation brought charges against France for taxing whisky and other grain-based alcoholic beverages more highly than cognac and grape-based beverages. French law requires a "purchase tax" on all alcoholic beverages based on alcohol content. The tax is applied in like fashion on both whisky and cognac. The French, however, differentiate between the two categories of alcohol by adding another tax called the "manufacturing tax" to grain-based aperitifs and other beverages, but the tax does not apply to grape-based "digestives" (Lubkin, 1996).

Because France is the world's leading producer of distilled wine (cognac), it had a great deal at stake. The court's ruling could change the balance of consumption between French cognac and British whisky. Britain is the world's largest producer of whisky.

The French defended their lower tax on grape-based alcohol because (1) cognac and whisky were not "similar" and (2) cognac and whisky did not compete for the same market. They also argued that grain-based whisky and grape-based cognac were made of different materials and were manufactured by different processes, resulting in products that tasted distinctly different (Lubkin, 1996).

The second argument was essentially a cultural appeal regarding the different uses of cognac and whisky in French daily life. According to the French, whisky was an "aperitif," to be drunk before dinner; cognac was a "digestive," to be drunk after dinner. In the social context, the cognac and whisky were not in competition and, the French claimed, would never drive consumers who sought an aperitif to purchase and drink cognac as a cheap alternative to whisky. Moreover the French argued that whisky consumption in France grew in the 1980s and 1990s at a rate about eight times faster than the rate of growth in cognac consumption (Lubkin, 1996).

Social Views, Customs, and Practices

The French people do not like to think of themselves as being hypocritical, a characteristic they typically associate with the British and Americans. This is one reason there is so much controversy over the use of cannabis. In 1998 French intellectuals began a discussion over the legitimacy of designating cannabis and hashish as soft drugs. Although such a debate in the United States would not have any effect on public or political thinking, in France it does. The French actually respect their intellectuals. Hence, in February 1998, 111 French artists and intellectuals signed a petition admitting to taking soft drugs and offering themselves up for prosecution. The intention was in part to embarrass the French government, but the main intent was to embarrass the French judiciary, which had prosecuted a number of high-profile drug campaigners who were working to reduce the legal penalties for using cannabis and other drugs. The signatories of the "petition of 111" include the 1960s Franco-German political activist Daniel Cohn-Bendit, the film director Patrice Chereau, the fashion designer and president of Paris Opera Pierre Berge, and the actress Marina Vlady. The petitioners state, "At one moment or other of my life, I have consumed stupefying drugs. I know that in admitting publicly that I am a drug user, I can be prosecuted. This is a risk I am ready to take" (Lichfield, 1998).

The motive was to draw attention to the hypocrisies and inconsistencies of the government's policy and the application of the French antidrug law. Admitting publicly to drug use can result in being prosecuted in France as an incitement to use by others. The president of Act-Up, a group campaigning for the legalization of soft drugs, was prosecuted for distributing a tract called "I Like Ecstasy" for breaking the same law. In another case, a counterculture newspaper, *L'Elephant Rose*, was forced into bankruptcy after being prosecuted under the incitement to use by others law. No legal action was taken against others, however, including pop singer Johnny Hallyday and Justice Minister Elisabeth Guignou, who have spoken openly about decriminalizing soft and hard drug use (Lichfield, 1998).

Treatment for Addiction in France

The underlying philosophy of treatment in France is that the addict is someone who uses drugs because he or she cannot cope with his or her circumstances. Likewise, treatment for the most part incorporates one of the standard forms of psychotherapy used in other countries such as the United States.

One thing is clear: Drug treatment excluding treatment for alcoholism has risen sharply in France since the 1980s. In view of France's financial and economic difficulties, several reforms have been implemented since the early 1980s to lower the cost of treatment. Another difference is that the medical profession in France is not directly involved in the regulation process of substance-abuse treatment as it is in Germany, and it is not in direct competition for treatment monies such as in the United States (Mossé, 1998).

Substance-abuse treatment in France did not really begin until the 1970s, and then it was viewed as an experimental phase. Physicians established treatment facilities on the margin of mainstream medicine. As treatment developed from the experimental to the more or less standard forms, it took on familiar characteristics. Participation in substance-abuse treatment is voluntary, and there is often a phase of detoxification followed by inpatient treatment or outpatient treatment. An annual report from the government itemizes the key attributes of patients treated during the year and the services they received. Statistics of the Ministry of Health and specialist organizations for 1994 put the number of visits to physicians or hospitals related to the abuse of drugs, excluding alcohol, to be over 100,000 visits. This number, in comparison to the total number of 250,000,000 visits and consultations for all illness, is insignificant. Statistics from hospitals in 1994 show that 40,000 drug users received inpatient treatment compared with a total of 15,000,000 inpatients. Both of these ratios suggest that only a relatively small percentage of drug users are treated in the health care system (Mossé, 1998).

Whereas market segmentation, the distribution of problem drug users within the social security and health-care systems, is already relatively advanced, the private and public sectors are split. The National Social Security system finances public and private care differently. Public hospitals are financed on a global budget, whereas private clinics continue to be funded on a per diem basis. Some of these clinics offer inpatient programs designed to reintegrate drug users into society after treatment. This is mainly offered to people between the ages of fifteen and thirty-five. For example, public hospitals offer inpatient care only to about 12 percent of the drug abusers they treat. In the private sector, this kind of care is offered almost exclusively. They provide 93 percent of all reintegration programs. In contrast, the public sector provides 75 percent of all withdrawal and detoxification services, and it is also where 75 percent of the drug users with AIDS, and 97 percent of those with other diseases, are primarily treated (Mossé, 1998).

The type of treatment often depends on whether it is to be mainly medical or mainly psychiatric. In general, detoxification follows several stages, beginning with five or six days without any drug substitution. Mainly in public hospitals, this phase may be shortened by medical intervention to accelerate the elimination of the drug. According to the seriousness of the withdrawal syndrome, a patient may be given a placebo instead of a substitution drug.

Despite this diversity, based mainly on a public and private divide, some professionals in the field believe that continuity of care is maintained because patients may be referred from one sector to the other according to their diagnoses, but there has been no systematic study to test this optimistic belief. Given the current distribution of patients between public and private services, economic incentives favor cooperation between ambulatory care, physicians, and inpatient facilities that treat the more severely affected drug users, but no such cooperation is apparent when social treatment is indicated. As such, public hospitals which accept the most seriously ill (who are most likely to be treated) must have a high turnover of patients, whereas the private facilities, which admit less severely affected patients, charge by the day and have an incentive to extend the length of stay.

THE FUTURE OF SUBSTANCE ABUSE IN FRANCE

Although French officials are nearing the point of giving into the pressure to accept that there is a difference between soft drugs and hard drugs, they are on the verge of changing their philosophical position on drug use. Many French people are coming to believe that the role of a progressive country is to protect their drug users by employing a health model to deal with the drug problem. For the French, this will be a major change in their moral view of drugs and drug users, particularly intravenous drug users.

French policy concerning harm reduction was nonexistent before the mid-1990s. By ignoring the irrational and conflicting drug policies, they became known as the "French syndrome" (Aeberhard, 1995). Even though it was a condescending characteristic, the enforcement of the former drug policies was no joke. The policies were responsible for violence, human rights abuses, and thousands of deaths. For that matter, the lack of knowledge, the prejudices, the misunderstandings, and the dogmatic certitude have indirectly killed thousands of heroin addicts throughout the world.

Proposed Solutions and Strategies

The economic crisis in the Western world in the mid-1990s created a new class of people—the so-called fourth world. This is the world of the homeless and the urban poor. The causes for these situations often differ from one developed country to another, but for those living in poverty, life is much the same throughout the fourth world. One policy that has been harmful to people living in these communities in France is the failure to provide methadone to heroin addicts. Ironically, in New York City, there are thousands of centers where drug addicts can obtain methadone, but clean needle-exchange programs were still illegal at the beginning of the twenty-first century. In France, methadone programs were rejected by the government and by most physicians, but clean needle-exchange programs were allowed.

One of the more novel approaches used in France to reduce the spread of HIV/AIDS is the vending machine that dispenses clean needles for used needles. These vending machines, introduced in Marseilles in 1996, were distributed in an attempt to reach a young group of intravenous drug users. A survey of intravenous drug users who obtained syringes from vending machines, pharmacies, and needle-exchange programs found that of the 343 users identified, 21.3 percent reported using vending machines as their primary source of syringes. Even more consequential, the primary users of the vending machines were more likely than other injection drug users to be younger than thirty years of age. They were less likely to have received drug maintenance treatment and to report not sharing needles or other drug-injection paraphernalia. These findings are particularly important since younger injection drug users are less likely to use needle-exchange programs and pharmacies as a source of sterile needles (Webster, 1999).

This study supports the concept that syringe vending machines can be a useful addition to other needle-exchange programs and to pharmacy sales of sterile syringes without prescription. However, whether the introduction of syringe vending machines is appropriate in other parts of France, or for that matter in other countries like the United States, is open to debate. Nonetheless, it does address part of the need to protect the health of high-risk young and short-term injection drug-using groups. Based on the data, the use of vending machines that dispense sterile syringes in communities with sizable intravenous drug users merits consideration.

CONCLUSION

France and the United States have a great deal in common in their approach to the drug war and drug users. In both countries, prohibition strategies have driven policy development. As a result, the French are faced with a fairly large number of heroin addicts—estimated at over 160,000. French officials continue to struggle with the widespread popularity and use of Moroccan hashish (Boekhout van Solinge, 1997). Heavy wine consumption at all ages is a serious problem, but it is not discussed openly. Of importance to a worldview of substance abuse, the spread of illegal drug use, abuse, and addiction in France has been described as mimicking an epidemic. First, like most epidemics, it attacked isolated minorities with whom the middle class did not identify. Second, when the epidemic reached into the middle class, it became a catastrophe and attracted a great deal of attention. Consequently, in the tragic case of the intravenous drug users who have died around the world of AIDS and who are HIV infected, we could observe that until their illness threatened to infect any one of us as well as any one of our children, we did not realize that by scorning the intravenous drug users we would end up scorning ourselves.

REFERENCES

Aeberhard, P.J. (1995). *The politics of harm reduction in France.* Paris: Médecins du Monde.

Boekhout van Solinge, T. (1997). Cannabis in France. In Lorenz Böllinger (Ed.), *Cannabis science. From prohibition to human right.* Frankfurt am Main: Peter Lang. Retrieved on December 1, 2000, from the World Wide Web: http://www.frw.uva.nl/cedro/library/Bremen95/France.html

Buck, J. (1997). Life in Languedoc. *Contemporary Review, 271,* 233–237.

Central Intelligence Agency. (2000). *The world factbook: France.* Washington, D.C.: prepared by the Central Intelligence Agency for the use of U.S. government officials. Retrieved November 20, 2000, from the World Wide Web: http://www.odci.gov/cia/publications/factbook/geos/fr.htm

Chabrol, H., Callahan, S., & Fredaigue, N. (2000). Cannabis use by French adolescents. *Journal of the American Academy of Child and Adolescent Psychiatry, 39 (4),* 400–401.

Encarta Desk Encyclopedia (1998). France. Microsoft Corporation on CD-ROM.

Epstein, E.J. (1977). *Agency of Fear: Opiates and Political Power in America.* New York: G.P. Putnam and Sons.

High committee report sheds new light on the state of health among French people. (1997). *The Globe.* Retrieved November 13, 2000, from the World Wide Web: http://www.ias.org.uk/theglobe/97issue1/

Institute of Alcohol Studies. (1997). *France—Country Profile.* London: Author. Retrieved November 26, 2000, from the World Wide Web: http://www.eurocare.org//profiles/France.htm

Korf, D.J., & Riper, H. (Eds.). (1997, November). Illicit drugs in Europe. *Proceedings of the Seventh Annual Conference on Drug Use and Drug Policy.* Amsterdam: Universiteit van Amsterdam, Faculteit der Rechtsgeleerdheid.

Lichfield, J. (1998, February). More than 100 French artists and intellectuals have signed a petition admitting to taking soft drugs and offering themselves for prosecution. *The Independent* (London), p. 1A.

Lubkin, G.P. (1996). *Is Europe's glass half-full or half-empty? The taxation of alcohol and the development of a European identity.* Cambridge, MA: Jean Monnet Chair of Harvard Law School.

Mossé, P. (1998). A system at its starting blocks: Drug treatment in France. In H. Klingemann, & G. Hunt, (Eds)., *Drug treatment systems in an international perspective: Drugs, demons, and delinquents* (pp. 201–209). Thousand Oaks, CA: Sage Publications.

U.S. Department of State (1999, March). *International Narcotics Control Strategy Report: Europe and Central Asia.* Washington, D.C.: Bureau for International Narcotics and Law Enforcement Affairs.

Webster, P. (1999, December 2). Syringe vending machines popular among young drug users. *Reuters Health*, p. 1A.

7

INDIA

Douglas Rugh

INTRODUCTION

India's traditional cultures have maintained many of their customary uses of alcohol and drugs. Both religious and secular reasons for using drugs have survived worldwide prohibition trends. This chapter explores some of these indigenous cultures with the hope of illuminating the population's beliefs and rationales for drug use in Indian society.

A Brief Profile of India

Union Minister of State for Health and Family Welfare Shri N.T. Shanmugam stated that India reached the one billion population mark on May 11, 2000. He claimed that India had reduced the crude birthrate from 40.8 in 1951 to 26.4 in 1998 and had halved the infant mortality rate from 146 per 1,000 live births in 1951 to 72 per 1,000 live births in 1998. Life expectancy has risen to sixty-two years from thirty-seven years in 1971 (Lexis-Nexis, 2000).

The people of India represent extreme diversities in language, religion, and socioeconomic class. Hindus account for 83 percent of the population and Muslims 11 percent (EIU, 1997). There are also Christians, Sikhs, Zoroastrians, Buddhists, Jains, and Jews. The total fertility rate in 1992 was 4 percent. Women make up 48.1 percent of the population (EIU, 1997). The sex ratio in rural India is 93 women to 100 men. This strong male bias is a result of infanticide, neglect of girls, and male migration to urban areas.

In 1992–93 only 9.2 percent of the households were headed by females (ESCAP, 1997).

In India, approximately 70 percent of the population earn their living from agriculture (EIU, 1997). Rural Indian girls and women are extensively involved in agricultural activities. Their roles range from managers to landless laborers. In overall farm production, the women's average contribution is estimated at between 55 and 66 percent of the total labor; the percentages are much higher in certain regions. In the Indian Himalayas, a pair of bullocks works 1,064 hours; a man, 1,212 hours; and a woman, 3,485 hours each year on a one-hectare (2.51 acres) farm (Venkateswaran, 1992).

The total adult illiteracy rate in India was 48 percent in 1995: 62 percent of women were illiterate, and 34 percent of men (UNDP, 1997). Both male and female literacy rates are substantially lower in rural areas than in urban areas. The difference between rural and urban rates is more pronounced in women. Rural females aged seven years and over are 30.4 percent literate, whereas the urban female population is 63.9 percent literate (ESCAP, 1997). These differences are important given that the rural population accounts for slightly more than 70 percent of the total population in India.

It is estimated that 42,000 babies are born every day in India. Four women, out of every 1,000, die giving birth—approximately forty women per day. In other words, every five minutes a woman dies because of a complication attributable to pregnancy or childbirth in India. It is estimated that, for each woman who dies, as many as thirty others develop chronic debilitating conditions that seriously affect their quality of life (Lexis-Nexis, 2000).

VIGNETTE

> Before you do anything, stop and recall the face of the poorest most helpless destitute person you have seen and ask yourself, "Is what I am about to do going to help him?"
>
> —Mahatma Gandhi

In the morning, smoke drifts up from the tea stall at the base of the buildings. The clay stove consists of a fiery oven bottom topped with a burner. A metal grating holds the coals. From below sticks of bamboo and scraps of wood are lit; no lighter fluid is used. The charcoal eventually ignites. The bent, blackened metal kettle holds about five gallons of water. The smells from the streets in the early morning and throughout the afternoon remind one of a fireplace.

Bullhorn speakers attached to long wooden poles emit fast paced screeches to wake the devout across the city. A small bundle of grasses tied at one end, which serves as a short broom, is used by one of the boys who hang around for odd jobs to sweep the front walkway. The boys squat until they are called upon to push the dirt into the dirty streets. Those on the way to the temple stop for a tea. Wooden benches line the walls and circle the vendors; as many as five sit on one bench.

Meanwhile, near the river, bathers wade into the water. Wooden funeral pyres burn nearby on the shore. The fires burn approximately twenty hours each day. The Indians who bathe in the Ganges River rapidly move their bodies in two ways. First, they throw their elbows backward, opening their chests and forcing deep breaths, and second they match their rapid breathing to a series of deep squatting knee bends. Old people travel to the banks of the Ganges for the honor of waiting to die.

Fried dough dipped in sugar syrup and milky sugar tea make the typical Indian breakfast. Most of the people in the streets have arrived in buses or packed auto rickshaws. They came in from the outlying village. The places skirting the city are as different from Varanasi as time and location allows. Fifty years, as well as ten kilometers, separate the city from the rural life. Later in the day, children sit in small groups where marbles smack together among the shouts.

I skirt the busy sections by dipping into the old part of the city. Here the streets turn into alleyways narrow enough that the cars and rickshaws cannot navigate the sharp turns. People walk and push bicycles. Water buffalo on their way from the banks to the shade of a tree force everyone to hug the walls of the buildings. These 900-year-old pathways are lined with belly-level shops. Customers step up to the shop floor, remove their shoes, and sit cross-legged with the merchant. He will show his silks, water heaters, cooking pots, jewelry, oils, perfumes, or whatever he happens to sell. Eventually, a young boy comes around with bhang, a sugary yogurt shake mixed with marijuana paste. The drink is used throughout the city as a way to relax through the long, hot afternoon. Bankers, policemen, and merchants of all types can be seen drinking a glass.

A warehouse factory sits on the top two floors of a building open to the air and directly in the middle of a residential area; this is a prime example of a tucked-away sweatshop. Obscure buildings conceal ten to fifteen hand-looms, where young boys and girls sit passing a shuttle back and forth. It's not a creative atmosphere; the looms are controlled with plastic punch cards designed to manipulate the weave in order to create a predetermined pattern. If the steps are followed, the brocade will be faithfully produced regardless of who sits at the loom. This seems to be Varanasi's largest industry. The guides tell me that silk has been made famous with its thousand-year history in the area.

Days end early in India. This environment slows people down since most things are out of reach. Crowded streets and slow rickshaws assure one that there is no use in rushing to do anything. The city simply will not allow it. The dropping sun starts to take on the appearance of a bright red planet.

As the sun drops, the light begins to travel through miles of dust: sand dust, road dust, and field dust. This causes a weak flaming red disc on the horizon. I can stare directly into it. The city takes on a magical aura during this time. Colors are enhanced, reds deepen to purple, blues darken. The streets do not slow as expected. Most shops stay open and the male energy increases. The movie area becomes even louder. The restaurants serve the crowds; the food smell works its way to the rooftops. The monkeys go home. Another group of Muslim chants are broadcast over the speaker system.

HISTORY OF SUBSTANCE ABUSE IN INDIA

Marijuana

A study conducted in Gulbarga and Belgaum, two districts of Karnataka in southern India, attempted to analyze drug abuse at the local and individual levels. The majority of the respondents in the study stated that the problem of drug abuse is not acute. It is confined to the use of ganja, or marijuana, which is seldom considered to be against the law. Many others are of the opinion that the cultivation and consumption of ganja have roots in customary practices. The study found that in a village sample, 161 out of 200 respondents used only ganja. Chewing ganja was reported by 32 respondents, and smoking it by 129. Eighty-nine respondents reported seasonal heavy use. For example, in Gulbarga, during the Holi festival, bhang (made from the leaves of *cannabis sativa*) and ganja are in great demand. Thirty-one respondents stated that ganja is used during marriages, and twenty reported medical use. All the respondents observed that ganja does not impede their work. None of the village respondents were drivers or industrial workers; however, they were predominantly involved in agriculture (140 respondents). Group consumption was seen as a matter of community practice by 144 of the respondents. Generally, during the ganja sessions, people discuss matters relating to family, marital, religious, and social functions (Joga Rao, 1994).

The question, "Why do they use ganja?," was answered in the following way. For 23 of them it is a family tradition, 24 use it for medicinal purposes, 29 use it because of religious beliefs, and 18 consider ganja good for the health. Another 117 respondents stated that consumption was a part of their life. According to 123 respondents, they have been consuming for a very long time, for more than ten years. With regard to prevention, 155 are of the opinion that it is not necessary. When queried about a stigma attached to ganja use, 56 responded negatively, 25 were not concerned about it, and only 17 indicated that ganja users are looked down upon. The majority of respondents (98) did not consider consumption to be antisocial, and 88 did not consider cultivation to be an antisocial activity (Joga Rao, 1994).

The question, "From where do they obtain their supplies?" was answered by the following response: a vast majority, 151 respondents, claimed that they obtain them directly from cultivators or by growing ganja plants. With regard to law enforcement, a majority of the respondents (111) are of the opinion that, for ganja, it is not necessary.

The following is a sampling of quotations from the report. "Ganja smoking is necessary to increase one's appetite"; "When the bride and bridegroom assemble for the ceremony of marriage, the bride's family is expected to distribute ganja to all the invitees—it is a well-known customary practice"; "In the festival of Saint Shishunal every devotee considers ganja smoking as a religious obligation"; "Chewing ganja helps us to get over anxiety and tiresomeness during work hours"; "Ganja smoking is a part of our day-to-day life" (Joga Rao, 1994).

The research report does not provide reliability and validity indicators or standardization of tools of data collection. However, based on the overwhelming evidence of culturally embedded use of ganja in the region, the following points should be noted. A thousand-year history of the use of cannabis cannot be wished away by national or international administrative fiats. Criminalization of cannabis can have massive implications for such cultures as those described above.

Opium

India is the world's largest producer of legal opiates for pharmaceutical purposes and the only country that still produces gum opium rather than concentrate of poppy straw (CPS). Opium is produced legally in the states of Madhya Pradesh, Rajasthan, and Uttar Pradesh.

There are no accurate data on the extent of opium and heroin addiction in India. The government estimates there are between one and five million opium users, and about one million heroin addicts throughout India, but some nongovernmental organizations estimate the number of addicts is much higher. The Ministry of Social Justice and Empowerment is now preparing to fund a comprehensive survey of narcotics addiction in India to be carried out by a contractor.

An addiction center at Veernagar, in the Rajkot district in the state of Gujarat, records 1,218 cases at the hospital from the years 1989/1990 to 1993/1994. The patients were users of crude heroin, alcohol, ganja (marijuana), or tobacco. Approximately 50 percent of them were opium addicts. Of the 607 opium addicts registered at the center, background information was available for 468. The description given below is based on the background data of these 468 opium addicts (Masihi, 1994).

All but one of the opium addicts were males. Seventy-eight percent were between thirty-six years of age and fifty-six years of age. They came from 207 villages in six districts of Saurashtra, that is, from almost all parts of Saurashtra. Opium addiction cuts across all castes. The upper castes (Brahmins, Bania, and Patidar,) constitute 12 percent of the addicts. The dominant castes (Rajput, Darbar, Kathis) comprise about 21 percent. All the other castes account for about 66 percent of the opium addicts. About 53 percent have been addicted to opium for the last ten years. Another 9 percent have been addicted for the last twenty years, and the rest (approximately 36 percent) for more than twenty years. In order to obtain a more detailed understanding of the current scenario of opium consumption, E.J. Masihi interviewed 158 opium consumers in twelve villages of six districts in the Saurashtra region (Masihi, 1994).

The 158 opium addicts were overwhelmingly males (two were females), and more than 53 percent were above fifty-six years of age; the mean age was 56.35 years. It is generally observed that opium addicts are older. A counselor noted, "An opium addict is accompanied by his son, whereas a brown sugar/heroin addict is accompanied by his father." In other words, heroin addicts are generally younger than opium addicts. The respondents were mostly Hindus (98.1 percent). Opium consumption was traditionally and culturally associated with the dominant caste and their subcastes in the region.

Contemporary opium drinkers come from all economic classes. Mud houses or huts constitute the dwellings of little more than half (53 percent) of the total. The majority (over 65 percent) is engaged in agriculture. Slightly less than one fourth (24 percent) are manual workers, and slightly over 8 percent are engaged in nonagricultural activities. Both joint and nuclear families consume opium. A joint family is defined as one in which husband and wife and their married children or any other relative stay in the home. The nuclear family is one in which only husband, wife, and their unmarried children stay. Respondents from joint families constitute about 10 percent of the total. About 89 percent are from nuclear families. About 11 percent are retired, and three were unemployed.

About 21 percent had started to use opium before the age of twenty-five. Somewhat less than half (48 percent) had started to use it between the ages of twenty-five and thirty-five. The rest had started after thirty-five years of age. The mean age is just over thirty-four years. The following four main reasons are given for using opium: friends were using it (67 percent), to alleviate sickness or disease (41 percent), to pass the time (34 percent), and to increase sexual potency (22 percent). Consumption by individuals devoid of company was not very popular in the past. Currently, because of the narcotics laws, consumption of opium in public is not very common. It was found that about 69 percent consume opium at home and alone. The rest consume with friends. The traditional practice of opium consumption was in the company of members of the same or a similar caste. That practice is no longer observed. The authors found that about 21 percent use opium with members of their own or members of other castes. The total number of friends consuming opium was quite large in the past. The size of the group has obviously decreased; most groups consist of two or three friends.

From the data, it was found that slightly more than 50 percent of the respondents take opium at least once daily. Those taking opium either three or two times a day constituted about 36 percent. The rest were taking it only occasionally during the week. It is not easy to obtain the required quantity. Thirty-two respondents, who cannot obtain opium, have switched over to opium pods. Those who consume opium use a maximum of 15 tolas (1 tola = 0.41 oz.) per week. Those who consume opium pods take a maximum of 7 oz. per week (it may be noted here that the research did not verify these figures by any established method). The practice of consuming opium on various other occasions, such as marriage and death, is also prevalent. Today opium is also consumed during election meetings, festivals, and events where a reconciliation takes place.

A majority of respondents (more than 58 percent) favor opium consumption in liquid form. About 33 percent consume it in the form of granules. Because of the difficulty in finding opium, a large number of respondents (90 percent) use opium pods soaked in water for about twelve hours. The water is then drunk. Permission to consume opium pods is given on medical grounds. It is also alleged that, during election time, contesting candidates help opium addicts to acquire permits for opium pods. About 47 percent of the respondents claimed to have such permits. However, many complained that they do not get enough pods even though they possess permits.

While opium drinkers historically ate rich food to help contain possible negative effects, only 26 of the respondents said that they take milk, ghee, eggs, and almonds after taking opium. More than one half (52 percent) of the respondents said that they could bear the expense of the habit. Of those who could not afford it, 36 percent had borrowed money, 11 percent had mortgaged their land, and 31 percent had sold their land or jewelry.

SOCIAL CONTEXT OF SUBSTANCE ABUSE

With India's relative isolation from western influences, it represents an excellent country to study the history of drug use with indigenous populations. Many ancient customs and rituals are still in practice today with little or no interference from international laws. This is starting to change after the Single Convention on Narcotic Drugs of 1961.

Alcohol

In India, most of the aboriginal people used to brew their own liquor made of rice, mahua flowers, or some other nutrient. Several macro changes have influenced the life of these people, leading to alcoholism on a wide scale. Industrialization, commercialization, westernization, and government policies have disenfranchised tribes from traditional resources. Land has become a marketable commodity. Through the promulgation of forest laws, restrictions have been introduced denying aboriginal people their traditional rights over the forest and its produce. In India, these people constitute about 9 percent of the population (approximately 900,000 people). Similarly, in Australia, Canada, and other countries, aboriginal people form a segment of the population that has been adversely affected by major social changes leading to alienation, hopelessness, and alcoholism.

The British introduced the policy of prohibiting aboriginal people from distilling liquor on their own to extract revenue from the tribes. They issued licenses for liquor shops, through auctions for the highest bidders. The alcohol became expensive to buy. Being removed of their cultural context, a sizable section of tribal society turned into addicts. The intensification of the process of alienation, deprivation of forestland, and dehumanization aggravated the problem of alcoholism in tribal society in most parts of the country. There were also attempts by social reformers to combat the consumption of alcohol. Followers of Mahatma Gandhi discouraged people from the use of alcohol with limited results. There were different mass movements against alcohol. For example, the Devi (goddess) movement, which spread in Gujarat and other areas, was fostered by individuals who, possessed by Devi, passed messages from village to village against alcohol consumption. This was part of a wider social reform movement against British influence and the trading class. The owners of liquor excise licenses steadily became property owners. This process occurred as liquor consumption gradually indebted the aboriginal people to the traders. This debt was paid off through the sale of tribal lands.

Opium

Opium consumption has several centuries of history in India. In Kashmir, it is smoked in groups; it is eaten in Punjab (where smoking is a religious taboo) and in Haryana. It is drunk in the desert regions of India in Gujarat and in Rajasthan. Administering opium to children to put them to sleep while the mothers work, during the teething period, and on other occasions for medicinal purposes is well documented (Britto, 1986; Modi, 1989; Shrivastava, 1989).

E.J. Masihi (1994) compiled data from secondary sources and reviewed relevant local literature on opium consumption in the Saurashtra region of Gujarat in western India. Opium forms part of the lifestyle of various segments of Saurashtra society. In the local language, opium was called *amal*, which means rule or control. Opium is consumed in two ways. Upper-caste people consume it in a liquid form. Opium is cut into small pieces and then ground to a paste with the help of a small, wooden pestle in a shallow mortar. The wooden pestle is made from the wood of the kerada tree, which is considered a cure for various ailments. Water is added to the paste. Other than opium, saffron or cardamom can be added. The liquid is then filtered several times through a thin cloth. Ultimately, when the required saffron (*kasumba*) color is reached, the liquid is either served in small metal vessels or in the cup of the palm. The type of vessels used to serve opium liquid reflect the economic and social status of the host. Opium-drinking gatherings, called *dayaro*, usually consist of men of the same or similar status. Women do not participate in such gatherings. The host pays for the opium consumed. Those present are usually his courtiers. Others could be a barber, a *charan* (religious leader), or a servant of the landlord. The barber prepares the liquid and serves it to the assembly. The *charan* regales the gathering with his songs. The *charan* is rewarded by the ruler or landlord for his songs of praise. The members of the gathering cannot refuse the opium liquid; to do so would insult the host. When opium liquid is served in the cup of a palm, the person can allow some of the liquid to flow out through his fingers. More than one serving is offered at a sitting. The *Kasumba Pani* is often followed by tea and rich snacks. It is necessary to take rich food to minimize the negative effects of the opium. Since the *dayaro* continues for many hours, only those men with enough leisure are in a position to take part. Those who had to earn their living each day took granules of opium to chew. This is called *rogu*.

In the past, several conditions provided an environment conducive to opium consumption. One is frequent battle. Warriors consumed opium to act as a painkiller when wounded. It was believed that opium increased strength to fight. It was also believed that opium had the capacity to increase sexual potency. Opium was part of the socialization process, and mothers gave it to their sons deliberately. Opium was used to cement friendship bonds. It was used as a mark of close friendship. At a time when restrictions on food and drinks were very severe and caste rules did not allow a man to accept food or water from members of other castes, the sharing of opium liquid was a mark of friendship and trust. That gesture converted enemies into friends, and opium was used to celebrate the event. On the other hand, opium was also used to ruin an enemy. It was considered the safest method of defeating an opponent. In extreme cases when people wanted to get away from any painful situation, they took an overdose of opium to end their lives. Women often resorted to it in case of domestic conflict.

The term opium has many names in the Charni dialect. It is called *afu*, *amal*, *galva*, *kanki*, *kasumbo* and *tijori*. Since opium was associated with warriors and ruling castes of Rajputs-Kathis, it was glorified in the oral literature. At the same time, there was another trend in the literature, wherein the negative side of opium was highlighted. However, the trend glorifying opium has remained more powerful than the negative one. *Charans* have used all their literary skills to glorify the drug.

A poet has said, "If the liquid is drunk by the father, his son gets the effect, if a horseman drinks it, the horse gets the effect. If an elephant drinks it, he becomes wild, if a cat tastes it, she can kill a tiger and likewise a donkey can kill an elephant, a dog can kill a lion and a sparrow can kill an eagle." Elsewhere opium is described as a companion of the traveler, a friend of the brave, and fire for the enemy. It is solace to the gloomy and a cure for the diseased. However, some local saints belonging to the Bhakti cult, as well as religious leaders of the Swaminarayan sect, preached against the use of opium. After pointing out various negative consequences of opium addiction, they declared that the intoxication of opium is only temporary, whereas the intoxication derived from devotion to God is permanent.

SUBSTANCE ABUSE IN INDIA TODAY

Political Views and Public Policies

India is an important producer of licit narcotics, some illicit narcotics, and is a crossroads for international narcotics trafficking. India is the world's largest producer of licit opium and the only producer of licit gum opium. The government of India continues to tighten controls to curtail diversion of licit opium to illicit markets. Nevertheless, an unknown quantity of opium is diverted from the country's legal production, and there is illegal poppy cultivation. Located between the two main sources of illicit opium, Southeast Asia and Southwest Asia, India is also a transit point for heroin, generally destined for Europe. There is little evidence to indicate that a significant quantity of illicit narcotics produced in or transiting through India reaches the United States. However, recent information points to the increased smuggling of ephedrine hydrochloride diverted from India's licit chemical industry to Mexican drug-trafficking organizations, which produce methamphetamine for the U.S. market.

The government supports drug-abuse treatment centers in 31 governmental medical institutions and 136 nongovernmental centers. A national federation of Indian nongovernmental organizations for drug-abuse prevention has been formed. Initiatives to reduce illicit drug demand include the development and implementation of a national strategy for community-based approaches and programs for the prevention of HIV and acquired immunodeficiency syndrome (AIDS).

Voluntary agencies conduct demand reduction and public awareness programs under grants from the Indian government. Despite increases in budget support for drug-abuse prevention and rehabilitation programs, which rose from approximately $1.5 million in 1991–1992 to $4.9 million in

1997–1998, this is inadequate given the extent of the problem. The government is developing drug rehabilitation and prevention programs in several major cities. Plans have been drawn to expand this program nationwide and to seek support from the corporate sector. In addition, the government of India has a comprehensive program for the northeastern states including de-addiction centers, training courses, and an awareness program. The government is now considering new initiatives to reduce illicit drug demand and reduce HIV/AIDS transmission through new community-based facilities. The Ministry of Social Justice and Empowerment also has established a center for drug-abuse prevention as part of the government's National Institute of Social Defense in New Delhi.

During 1998 the National Institute on Drug Abuse (NIDA, part of the U.S. National Institutes of Health) sponsored a workshop on drug abuse in Chennai and funded travel to conferences in the United States on demand reduction and the reduction of HIV risk among drug abusers. NIDA also initiated a United States–India Fund (USIF) research project on intravenous drug users and HIV prevention in New Delhi. In June 1998 the director of NIDA met with the Indian minister of state for social justice and empowerment in New Delhi on demand-reduction programs. In 1998 the U.S. Information Service (USIS) funded demand-reduction training seminars in Jaipur and New Delhi in cooperation with the Indian Psychiatric Society and the Jawaharlal Nehru University and sent a professor of psychiatry from the All India Institute of Medical Sciences to the United States for a program on substance-abuse prevention and education.

The government took a number of steps in the past several years to address what it conceded are serious shortcomings in its licit opium cultivation program. It first concentrated on improving factory and inventory security. In 1997 it turned its attention to collecting the harvested opium gum into government warehouses, with a sharp increase in the realized 1997 harvest. In the coming years, the United States plans to encourage the government of India to ensure an adequate supply of licit opium; intensify its efforts to combat illicit cultivation and trafficking; improve its extradition practices; identify, prosecute, and convict corrupt officials; and pass enabling legislation in support of the 1988 United Nations Drug Convention (*International Narcotics Control Strategy Report*, 1999).

Social Views, Customs, and Practices

The changes in drug-abuse trends in South Asia continue: in Bangladesh, India, and Nepal, the drug of abuse is shifting from opium to heroin and, more recently, also to buprenorphine, a potent synthetic opioid manufactured in India. The route of administration is shifting from inhalation (smoking) to injection. The abuse of codeine-based cough syrups has taken on substantial proportions in several parts of the region. The increase in the abuse of opioids (buprenorphine and codeine) has been facilitated by weaknesses in the controls over the licit drug supply system. Pharmaceutical preparations containing narcotic drugs or psychotropic substances are available without medical prescription. Despite strengthened regulatory and control measures and significant law enforcement successes, the illicit manufacture of methaqualone and the smuggling of that substance onto the world market continues.

Licit opium poppy cultivation and opium production are under governmental control in India. Some diversion has occurred in the opium production areas; consequently, controls over cultivation and production have been strengthened and licenses of farmers not complying with regulations have been withdrawn. The number of licensed farmers for the crop year 1995–1996 has decreased from 104,000 to 78,000.

Indian authorities have detected and destroyed a number of laboratories manufacturing crude heroin. In 1995 there was an increase of more than 50 percent in the total amount of heroin seized in India, while the amount of seized heroin originating in Southwest Asia increased by over 300 percent.

THE FUTURE OF SUBSTANCE ABUSE IN INDIA

In India, traditional abuse of opium still continues in some provinces, but in many others the abuse of heroin or synthetic opioids is increasing. There have been continuing reports on an alarming increase in opiate dependence in the northeastern part of the country, which borders the opium-producing areas of Southeast Asia. Inhalation is the most frequent route of administration used by heroin abusers in Bangladesh, Nepal, and Sri Lanka; however, in India there are signs of increased use of injection, a major factor contributing to the spread of HIV infection among drug abusers in that country.

In Bangladesh, India, and Nepal, the large-scale abuse of cough syrups continues. Because of weaknesses in the controls over the pharmaceutical supply system, a number of genuine, counterfeit, and fake syrups are freely available in those countries. Reports on the composition of these preparations have been contradictory, but codeine phosphate is usually the main ingredient. The reports also contradict each other concerning the codeine content of the preparations.

Despite the efforts of competent authorities, the illicit manufacture of methaqualone continues in India. In 1995 four clandestine laboratories were destroyed, and twenty tons of methaqualone were seized. Substantial amounts of methaqualone were smuggled out of India into eastern and southern Africa. Control of the important methaqualone precursor N-acetylanthranilic acid and increased law enforcement measures have resulted in a reduction of clandestine manufacturing activities in the Bombay area.

However, it is feared that such activities might simply have shifted to elsewhere within or outside India.

CONCLUSION

Traditionally, drugs were used in a crude form and were mostly eaten, though smoking of opium and cannabis drugs was quite common. This type of use is shifting as India fully engages the world economic markets, and along with this shift will come more purified, higher priced forms of drugs. As India continues to industrialize and thereby build its wealth, alcohol and drugs will play an increasingly important role in India's economy.

REFERENCES

Britto, G., et al. (1986). *Policy perspectives in the management of drug abuse in India.* Bombay: Society for the Promotion of Area Resource Centres, National Addiction Research Network.

Bureau for International Narcotics and Law Enforcement Affairs, U.S. Department of State, Southwest Asia. (1999). *International narcotics control strategy report.* Washington, D.C.: U.S. Department of State. Downloaded on November 11, 2000, from http://www.usis.usemb.se/drugs/1998.html

Charles, M., Masihi, E.J., Siddiqui, H.Y., Jogarao, S.V., D'lima, H., Mehta, U., Britto, G. (1994). Culture, drug abuse and some reflections on the family (pp. 67–86). National Addiction Research Centre, Bombay, India.

EIU. (1997). *India Nepal: Country Profile.* London: The Economist Intelligence Unit.

ESCAP. (1997). *Women in India: A country profile.* New York: United Nations.

Joga Rao, S.V. (1994). *Culture and cannabis in rural Karnataka.* Unpublished manuscript, National School of Law, India University and National Addiction Research Center, Bombay.

Lexis-Nexis. (2000). Indian government national population policy 2000 on Web site. M2 Communications Ltd., M2 Presswire, May 11, 2000.

Masihi, E.J. (1994). *Culture, drug use and abuse: A case-study of opium consumption in Saurashtra.* Paper presented at the International Symposium on Culture, Ahmedabad, India.

Mehta, U. (1994, January). *Culture and drug abuse in Dang.* Paper presented at the International Symposium on Culture, Drug Use and Abuse in Asian Settings, Bangkok, Thailand.

Modi, I.P. (1984). *Assessment of drug abuse, drug users and drug prevention services in Ajmer.* New Delhi: Ministry of Welfare, Government of India.

Shrivastava, R.S. (1989). *An assessment of drug abuse, drug users and drug prevention services in the city of Jodhpur.* New Delhi: Ministry of Welfare, Government of India.

UNDP. (1997). *Human Development Report.* New York: Oxford University Press.

Venkateswaran, S. (1992). *Living on the edge: Women, environment and development.* New Delhi: Friedrich Ebert Stiftung.

8

IRELAND

Mary E. Dillon

INTRODUCTION

According to a lament in a popular Irish song, "Ireland is a land of happy wars and sad love songs." This may be somewhat true, but the history of the Irish, and subsequently the history of Irish Americans, is tied to the stigma associated with heavy alcohol consumption. Drugs such as Ecstasy are a recent phenomenon among the youth in the larger cities of Ireland. However, even among the young, alcohol abuse continues to be the major concern.

The drinking of alcohol is an integral part of Irish social life, and it is accepted as such by most Irish people. It plays an important role in social, cultural, and sporting activities. However, alcohol is also a drug (British Medical Association, 1991), which while used and enjoyed by many people, has led to significant problems both for the individual and for the community at large when it is taken to excess, or when the user becomes addicted to alcohol. The misuse of alcohol can result in harm to physical and emotional health, in economic loss, in violence and disruption of family life, and in the maiming and killing of the drinker and others in accidents, especially automobile accidents (National Roads Authority, 1994).

In a recent report published by the National Alcohol Policy Agency of Ireland, it has been anticipated that alcohol consumption will continue to increase in the Irish population in the coming years (Conniffe and McCoy, 2001), given the current and projected economic growth. It is anticipated there will be an increase in the number of people drinking beer because it is less sensitive to price increases. There are increasing exemptions for longer opening hours of premises that serve alcohol. Clearly, a greater number of young people are starting to drink beer at a younger age. There is a higher percentage of regular drinkers by the age of eighteen years with a preference for beer than there was in the early 1980s. There are increased alcohol advertising campaigns in the media in terms of volume, exposure, and extensive sponsorship promotions with highly visible sports (ASAI, 1995).

The role that Ireland plays in alcohol and other drug consumption in the European Union (EU) and its implications for treatment and policy issues around the world are important for understanding issues related to substance abuse in the new millenium.

A Brief Profile of Ireland

To give an accurate profile of Ireland, we must divide the island into two separate entities: the Republic of Ireland and Northern Ireland.

Ireland was first inhabited around 7500 B.C. by Mesolithic hunter-fishers, probably from Scotland. They were followed by Neolithic people, who used flint tools, and then by people from the Mediterranean, known in legend as the Firbolgs, who used bronze implements. Later came the Picts, also an immigrant people of the Bronze Age. During the Iron Age, the Celtic invasion (around 350 B.C.) introduced a new cultural strain into Ireland, one that was to predominate. The oldest relics of the Celtic language can be seen in the fifth-century Ogham stone inscriptions in county Kerry. Ireland was Christianized by Saint Patrick in the fifth century. The churches and monasteries founded by him and his successors became the fountainhead from which Christian art and refinement permeated the crude and warlike Celtic way of life (Dietler, 1994).

The Republic of Ireland

This region comprises about five-sixths of the island of Ireland. The country consists of the provinces of Leinster, Munster, and Connacht and part of the province of Ulster. The rest of Ulster, which occupies the northeastern part of the island, constitutes Northern Ireland. The Irish Republic has an area of 70,273 square kilometers (27,133 square miles). The capital of the Republic of Ireland is Dublin. The population of the Irish Republic is predominantly of Celtic origin. The Celts were some of the earliest people on the island, the prehistoric people known as Iberians. The Celts tended to be shorter than their Anglo-Saxon counterparts. Most had darker hair, but a strikingly high percentage of Celts had red hair.

The population of the Irish Republic in 1998 was estimated at 3,619,480, giving the country an overall population density of 52 persons per square kilometers (133 per square mile). The population decreased from the 1840s, when about 6.5 million people lived in the areas included in the republic, until about 1970, largely because of a high emigration rate. During the 1980s the population increased at an annual rate of only about 0.5 percent, and by 1998 the rate had slowed to 0.36 percent. Some 58 percent of the population lived in urban areas in 1997.

Northern Ireland

Northern Ireland, an integral part of the United Kingdom of Great Britain and Northern Ireland, is situated in the northeastern portion of the island of Ireland. Northern Ireland is bounded on the north and northeast by the North Channel, on the southeast by the Irish Sea, and on the south and west by the Republic of Ireland. Northern Ireland is also known as Ulster, because it comprises six of the nine counties that constituted the former province of Ulster. The total area of Northern Ireland is 14,160 square kilometers (5,470 square miles). In Northern Ireland, the majority of the people are of Scottish or English ancestry and are known commonly as the Scotch-Irish. The remainder of the population is Irish, principally native to Ulster. In 1996 the estimated population of Northern Ireland was 1,663,000. The overall density was about 11 persons per square kilometer (about 28 per square mile). The population is unevenly distributed, with greater concentrations in the eastern half. It is almost equally divided between urban and rural dwellers. The capital of Northern Ireland is Belfast (population estimate, 296,700), which is surrounded by heavy industries including shipbuilding and textiles. The other major city in Northern Ireland is Londonderry (which is called "Derry" by the Irish population).

Land and Resources

In the Republic of Ireland the eastern coast of Ireland is fairly regular with few deep indentations; the western coast is fringed by drowned or submerged valleys, steep cliffs, and hundreds of small islands torn from the mainland mass by the powerful forces of the Atlantic Ocean. Numerous bogs and lakes are found in the lowland regions. The principal rivers of Ireland are the Erne and the Shannon, which are actually chains of lakes joined by stretches of river. All of Ireland's principal rivers flow from the plain, and an interior canal systems facilitates transportation.

Northern Ireland has an extreme northern to southern extension of about 135 kilometers (about 85 miles) and an extreme eastern to western extension of about 175 kilometers (about 110 miles). The shoreline, which is characterized by numerous irregularities, is about 530 kilometers (about 330 miles) long. The major indentations are Lough Foyle in the north and Belfast, Strangford, and Carlingford loughs in the east. A striking feature of the northern coast is the Giant's Causeway, a rock formation consisting of thousands of closely placed, polygonal pillars of black basalt. The chief rivers are the Boyne River, which forms part of the northwestern boundary and flows into Lough Foyle at Londenderry, and the Upper Bann and Lower

Bann rivers. The former rises in the Mourne Mountains and empties into Lough Neagh; the latter flows out of Lough Neagh to the North Channel. Among the many other rivers are the Main, Blackwater, Lagan, Erne, and Bush. Because of the generally flat terrain, drainage is poor, and the areas of marshland are extensive.

Climate

The climate of the Republic of Ireland and Northern Ireland are very similar and are like those of other islands. Because of the moderating influence of prevailing warm, moist winds from the Atlantic Ocean, the mean winter temperature ranges from 4° to 7°C (40° to 45°F), approximately 14°C (25°F) higher than that of any other place in the same latitude in the interior of Europe or on the eastern coast of North America. The oceanic influence is also pronounced in the summer; the mean temperature of Ireland ranges from 15° to 17°C (59° to 62°F), about 4°C (7°F) lower than that of other places in the same latitudes. Rainfall averages 1,000 millimeters (40 inches) annually.

Religion and Language

In the Irish Republic, Catholics make up to 93 percent of the people of Ireland, and 4 percent are Protestants. Protestant groups include the Church of Ireland (Anglican) and the Presbyterian and Methodist denominations. Freedom of worship is guaranteed by the constitution.

Almost all the people speak English, and about one-fourth also speak Irish, a Gaelic language that is the traditional tongue of Ireland. Irish is spoken as the vernacular by a relatively small number of people, mostly in areas of the west. The constitution provides for both Irish and English as official languages.

Religious affiliation has been a key determinant in Northern Ireland's history, politics, and social life since its beginning. At various times it has determined access to voting and jobs, standards of living, and education. In modern times, it has come to symbolize the differences between the descendants of the original inhabitants and those of the settler community. The descendants of the Scottish and English settlers are predominantly Protestant; those of the original Irish inhabitants are overwhelmingly Roman Catholic. In the early 1990s, almost 51 percent of the population regarded themselves as Protestant, and almost 39 percent as Roman Catholic. The Roman Catholics are the largest single denomination. The largest Protestant denominations are the Presbyterians, the Church of Ireland, and the Methodists. Unlike England, Northern Ireland has no established, or state, church. The Church of Ireland, at one time a branch of the Church of England, was disassociated from the state in 1871.

Education

Irish influence on Western education began fourteen centuries ago. From the sixth to the eighth century, when Western Europe was largely illiterate, nearly 1,000 Irish missionaries traveled to England and the Continent to teach Christianity. During the early Middle Ages, Irish missionaries founded monasteries that achieved an extensive cultural influence.

Classical studies flowered in ancient Ireland. Distinctive also at the time were the bardic schools of writers and other learned men who traveled from town to town, teaching their arts to students. The bardic schools, an important part of Irish education, were suppressed in the sixteenth century by King Henry VIII of England.

In what is now the Republic of Ireland, university education began with the founding of the University of Dublin, or Trinity College, in 1592. In Northern Ireland, Queen's University was founded in 1845.

Both the Irish Republic and Northern Ireland have a free public school system. In the Irish Republic, compulsory education is provided for all children between the ages of six and fifteen; in Northern Ireland, education is free and compulsory to children between the ages of four and sixteen (*Encarta Desk Encyclopedia*, 1998).

Economy

The economy in the Republic of Ireland has been traditionally agricultural. Since the mid-1950s, however, the country's industrial base has expanded, and now mining, manufacturing, construction, and public utilities account for 36 percent of the gross domestic product (GDP), while agriculture accounts for only about 10 percent. Private enterprise operates in most sectors of the economy. The GDP in 1997 was $75 billion.

The GDP of Northern Ireland in 1992 was about $18.3 billion. In general, the economy of Northern Ireland is based on agriculture and manufacturing and is closely tied to that of Britain as a whole; almost half of manufacturing output is sold to the rest of Britain; one quarter is sold locally. Northern Ireland has been particularly hard hit by the decline of traditional industries like shipbuilding, on which much of its prosperity and many jobs depended. The lack of economic opportunities, particularly for young people, played a role in the sectarian conflicts of the 1970s. At the same time, however, the threat of terrorism hindered efforts to attract investments and decreased new jobs in the 1990s. Considerable public expenditure has been devoted to urban renewal in Belfast and Londonderry. Various agencies have been established to attract new companies and encourage small businesses, backed by tax and other incentives. Helped by moves toward a peaceful settlement of the sectarian violence, several important new investments were announced in the early 1990s. Public finance came predominantly from taxes (50 percent in 1994) and government grants in aid from the United Kingdom (41 percent). Northern Ireland also receives considerable funding from the European Union.

VIGNETTE

Seamus Crowley lived in the remote farming community of Ballyblue in the western part of the Republic of Ireland. Seamus Crowley and his wife Maggie had six children, ranging in ages from sixteen to four years old. Mary Crowley was the oldest and was the one who worked the hardest as a part-time housekeeper. Mary excelled in her studies in school. Maggie Crowley experienced three miscarriages after the births of her six children, and there would have been more children, but a hysterectomy had dramatically terminated Maggie Crowley's years of fertility.

Seamus Crowley was recognized by all as a good-for-nothing, although his worst enemies would agree that he was good for fathering children and for "wheedling" drinks. It was an occupation at which Seamus Crowley had become an expert. He learned over the years that even the most unlikely sources could sometimes show a profitable return with little effort when it came to the drink.

At one of the local pubs Seamus sat on a high stool, surveying the crowd that may produce another drink. He thought "fat chance" as all the other imbibers were recipients of the social welfare like himself and would argue that they had no more than enough to satisfy their own needs. One Guarda (policeman) remarked that "all the farmers do all the work, and the unemployed do all the drinking!"

Mary Crowley was a product of an abusive, alcoholic father. Her mother and other siblings had to hide outside the house when their father came home drunk. If not, they would be subjected to severe physical and mental abuse. The result of living in this abusive atmosphere led to circumstances in Mary's life that turned tragic.

Mary met a boy named Johnnyboy at school; his parents were the proprietors of the local supermarket. Of all their three boys, Johnnyboy was the least likable and most selfish of the lot. On several occasions, Johnnyboy waited for Mary to complete her housekeeping duties in the countryside and walked her home. After he asked her to a local school dance, he brought along poteen, the American equivalent of moonshine or white lightning, which has an alcohol level in excess of 150 proof. Mary became intoxicated and Johnnyboy took advantage of her sexually, another byproduct of alcohol abuse. When Mary found out she was pregnant she was frantic and needed to talk to her mother.

One night before her father arrived home from the local pub, Mary confronted her mother in the kitchen of their home. Mary said, "Mother I need to talk to you." Maggie Crowley looked hard and long at her daughter's pinched face before denying her request. Maggie said, "I don't want to talk to you Mary. I don't want to hear anything that will make the cross I'm carrying any heavier. I don't want your father laying the pair of us out cold on the floor of this kitchen. I'll talk to you some other time Mary, but not now." This statement was accompanied by a look of terror on her mother's face as she heard the approach of Seamus Crowley.

Without counsel of her mother, Mary became so despondent that one night after her housekeeping duties she walked to the River Moy and sat down. Sensing that her father in an alcoholic rage would beat her to death when he found out about her pregnancy, she chose the only option open to her at the time. She walked into the River Moy until the current took her away from all her troubles.

After Mary's death, the older boys became less tolerant of their father's drunken binges and subsequent beatings of themselves and their mother. They took drastic measures.

After spending an hour at Mary Crowley's grave saying the Rosary, the two oldest Crowley boys asked their mother and sisters to go to Tom's Tavern for a sandwich and a drink. Soon, Seamus Crowley noticed his family's presence in the local pub. He stormed in and asked where they obtained the money to eat and drink in the pub. The two oldest boys stated that they had earned the wages that day. Seamus became outraged and dragged the two boys outside where he proceeded to beat them. When Maggie emerged, she leapt on Seamus's back and started to take him down while in his drunken stupor.

The humorous part of this true tale is that it did not take an addiction recovery center or AA to cure Seamus of his alcoholic problems; it took a physical threat to make him mend his ways.

After Seamus was shut out of his house for several days, the local parish priest tried to intervene with Maggie Crowley, saying that Seamus had repented and wanted to come home. However, it was not divine intervention or AA who saved Seamus; it was the local proprietor of Tom's Tavern who told Seamus Crowley that "he would never again indulge in strong drink, he would find a job and provide for his wife and family, and he would never raise a hand to his wife or any of his offspring ever again." The threat went on to state that if he did drink "he would be taken from his abode, a block of limestone tied to his neck and from the loftiest cliff-bank on the river Moy would be cast without ceremony unto the deepest hold, there to disintegrate until the day of judgement when the angel Gabriel would blow his horn to summon the living and the dead!"

Seamus observed the conditions and although the people of Ballyblue marvelled at the transformation that took place, they never knew the why and the whereof, except that Seamus took to polishing his shoes and wearing clean shirts as well as being civil to his neighbors, loving to his wife and family, and living in the fear of God, late in the day though it might be. Whatever the somewhat positive ending, Seamus Crowley lost a daughter and a grandchild, all as a result of the "drink."

SUBSTANCE ABUSE IN IRELAND AND BASIC DEMOGRAPHICS

The Irish National Alcohol Policy was launched in 1996. The main policy objective was to promote moderation in alcohol consumption, for those who wish to drink, and to reduce the prevalence of alcohol-related problems in Ireland. The plan of action in the policy sets out the required actions to be taken by the different partners, such as government departments, health boards, and the drinks industry, to bring about effective implementation.

According to the 1997 report, *Ireland—Overview Report on Alcohol* published by the Institute of Alcohol Studies, there has been a steady increase in alcohol consumption in Ireland since the late 1980s. In 1990, the average consumption of alcohol for those over the age of fifteen was 2.4 gallons per person. In 1996, the consumption rate rose to 3.2 gallons.

HISTORY OF ALCOHOL AND DRUG ABUSE IN IRELAND

In the late eighteenth and nineteenth centuries, drinking behavior and attitudes in England, Scotland, Ireland, and Northern Europe were quite similar in that drinking rituals were part of a typical workday of every occupation and profession. Since Ireland lacked a substantial middle class, hard drinking did not become taboo. Instead, it was a way of coping with economic hardships (Conniffe and McCoy, 2001).

British land reform gave Irish Catholics the opportunity to own land. This allowed families to consolidate their holdings. However, the Great Famine in the 1800s ended minute subdivision of land.

Marriage now was tied to ownership of land. As such, this created a large class of unmarried men and women. Although many migrated to the United States, those who stayed in Ireland married late after their parents gave them the land, and a new pattern of few and late marriages was created. Bachelor groups emerged with emphasis on sports, fighting, storytelling, and hard drinking, which became the rites of passage to adulthood.

Historically, drunkenness was different than hard drinking. If you could hold your own, hard drinking was acceptable. Most people felt that hard drinkers were the bulwark of the community. Hence, it was perceived that it was better to permit hard drinking and even occasional drunkenness than to risk the possibility of early marriage or illegitimacy, which would threaten the economic order. In other words, it was better to drink than to threaten the system. Emphasis upon chastity and related prohibitions against birth control and abortion compounded the problem. Illegitimacy was not only sinful according to the Catholic Church, it threatened the new family farm economy, which linked marriage and land ownership.

SUBSTANCE ABUSE IN IRELAND TODAY

The Health Strategy Documents of 1994 and 1995 contain recommendations concerning the development of a National Alcohol Policy, and in 1996 the National Alcohol Policy was published. This policy was directed at encouraging moderation for those who choose to drink, and reducing the prevalence of alcohol-related problems. As in previous strategy documents, the importance of a multisectoral approach to health promotion initiatives was stressed. It was postulated that an awareness and understanding of the National Alcohol Policy and how it should be implemented in respective areas of responsibility could create an effective support network.

There is a growing body of research and expertise in Ireland in the range of issues involved in alcohol dependency. Trinity College recently established an addiction research center, a collaborative venture between the Department of Social Studies and the School of Pharmacy, with the aim of providing a source for competent, independent, and critical research into the prevention management of alcohol and drug problems in Ireland. This additional research and training should dramatically help in setting up effective treatment services.

Political Views and Public Policies

Consumers do not generally organize into groups that raise strong and unified voices in the political arena. Nonetheless, they have opinions that can be measured by opinion polls, and they cast the ballots that elect the politicians who make social and economic policy. Steep rises in any taxes are rarely popular with consumers, especially when it comes to alcohol taxation.

At the other end of the political spectrum, on the subject of alcohol, taxation is the interest represented by temperance advocates. Since that interest is moral and not economic, the level of taxation tends to be of less interest to them than the strict regulation, or total prohibition, of consumption opportunities. Temperance advocates have a voice in some parts of Europe, especially in the northern member states, but they have little direct influence in setting tax policy. However, it is probably not coincidental that Ireland, the member state with the highest percentage of its revenue derived from alcohol excise taxation, is also the member state with the highest percentage of "teetotallers" in its population (European Commission, 1993).

The cost of alcohol has an important influence on consumption levels, and it is subject to the economic laws of supply and demand. The effect of price changes on alcohol consumption has been extensively investigated in Western societies such as North America, Australia, New Zealand, and Europe. The extent of the findings is that if alcohol prices go up consumption goes down, and if prices go down consumption goes up (Edwards, 1994). However, there is greater price sensitivity in spirits and wine than in beer consumption, and this is especially evident in English-speaking countries (Edwards, 1997).

Excise taxes in general have a practical appeal to governments. These indirect levies can be applied to specific target commodities with great flexibility. Rates in particular can be changed from year to year in response to current revenue requirements, policy shifts, and public opinion. In 1992, the last year before frontier controls were removed under the single market, the percentage of total excise taxes derived from alcohol ranged from as low as 2 percent in Italy to as high as 27 percent in Ireland (Coopers and Lybrand, 1994, p. 14).

Excise taxes are appealing to governments not only as a revenue source, but also as a convenient mechanism for promoting other policy purposes. The three most heavily excised commodities are alcohol, tobacco, and mineral oils (Coopers and Lybrand, 1994, p. 15). Adjusting excise taxation on any of these commodities can discourage consumption, encourage preference of one form or application of the product over another, and pay the costs of externalities associated with the use of that commodity, such as treatment.

One interesting contradiction in substance abuse among the youth, and the population in general, is the price differential between soft drinks and alcoholic beverages. This caused a major concern in the general population. The concern was that the prices of soft drinks in on-licensed premises was so high as to make them not competitive with alcoholic drinks, which may discourage people from substituting nonalcoholic drinks for alcoholic drinks (Morgan and Grube, 1994).

Social Views, Customs, and Practices

In researching the literature on Ireland, it is apparent that the psychiatric hospital model for treatment seems to be the norm. The aim of treatment services in Ireland for alcohol dependence is to help individuals end their dependence on alcohol and to rebuild relationships with their spouses, families, friends, and colleagues. For those whose dependence has progressed to the stage that they have become homeless and destitute, the services they require are shelter, care, and treatment for the physical and mental illnesses associated with advanced alcohol dependence.

The psychiatric model in Ireland has had its controversy over time. The appropriateness of the psychiatric hospital model of treatment for alcohol dependence came under scrutiny in Ireland in the 1970s. The Report on the Development of Psychiatric Services, *Planning for the Future*, recommended in 1984 that alternative community-based services be developed. *The Green Paper on Mental Health*, published by the government in June 1992, comments that in the years since publication of *Planning for the Future*, some health boards have developed local alcohol and drug services and recruited addiction counselors to work in sector services. It also pointed to the extremely high rate of admission to psychiatric hospitals for alcohol-related disorders in some health boards and suggests that such rates demonstrated the need to develop alternative treatment facilities in the community (Nic Gabhainn and Kelleher, 1995).

In Ireland, apparently there is no one alcohol treatment program that is clearly more effective than another. The lack of any vigorous evaluation of the outcome of treatment in different settings and using different therapies makes it difficult to provide a firm basis for recommendations. However, the present state of knowledge suggests that outpatient models of treatment are no less effective than inpatient care, yet they have the advantage of being less expensive. Today, the main therapeutic tools in the treatment of alcohol dependency are psychotherapy, counseling, family and marital therapy, either individually or in group settings.

In the treatment models presented, support for families with an alcohol-dependent spouse, who may experience many physical, psychological, and social problems, requires different levels of support, and from a variety of sources, such as the family general practitioner, schools, and social workers. An important group to recognize is children who are at high risk of alcohol or drug consumption and may require specific counseling.

THE FUTURE OF SUBSTANCE ABUSE IN IRELAND

It has become alarming in recent years that Ireland has the highest rate of drug-related deaths in the EU. The average age for Dublin youth, for example, to take their first drink is eleven, and 14 percent have abused inhalants, such as glue. It was also reported that youths in Northern Ireland, between the ages of fourteen and twenty, started using alcohol before they were 14.5 years old. They started using soft drugs before they were sixteen years old, and they started using hard drugs six months after using soft drugs. The real story in these numbers, however, even more alarming, is the lifetime prevalence of soft drugs among Northern Ireland's females between fourteen and twenty: 33.4 percent (McDonald, 1997). For the boys of the same age, it is 17.8 percent. This is one of the highest rates among a group of young people on record. There is no national data available on any country that shows girls have a higher lifetime prevalence on soft and hard drug use as compared to boys (See Figure 8.1).

When girls use soft drugs at twice the rate of their male counterparts, something is desperately wrong. In this case, the environment in Northern

Figure 8.1
Lifetime Prevalence of Use of Both Hard and Soft Drugs by Youth between Fourteen and Twenty Years of Age by Gender

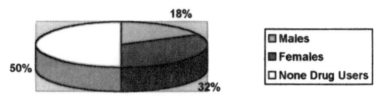

Ireland in the year 2000 is unstable, and the future for Northern Ireland's youth is in question. These environmental characteristics coalesce to increase the need for release of emotional uncertainty.

The future of alcohol and drug abuse in Ireland lies with its future leaders—its youth of today. The greatest single concern voiced in submissions from the public concerned problems associated with teenage access to alcohol (O'Kelley, 1999).

The importance of early intervention to change drinking patterns that are associated with alcohol dependency underlines the role of the health-care professions in dealing with the problem. The general practitioner is instrumental in advising the population on sensible drinking and in connecting presenting signs and symptoms related to alcohol dependence. The Irish College of General Practitioners (ICGP, 1991) has recommended that general practitioners be proactive in the education, identification, diagnosis, and treatment of patients with alcohol-related problems.

Proposed Solutions and Strategies

It is apparent that there are three areas in which the alcohol industry makes a significant contribution to the Irish economy: employment, revenue by taxes, and balance of payments. The alcohol industry is a positive contributor to Ireland's balance of payments with the value of alcohol exports being nearly three times that of imports in 1991 (Department of Health and Children, 1996). But what is the cost?

It is important to note that a multisectoral approach to health promotion was highlighted in the 1995 Health Promotion strategy document. Professionals and voluntary groups in both the health and other sector areas can make a significant contribution to the health and social gain of the community.

This can be accomplished by influencing people's attitudes and habits so that, for those who choose to drink, moderate drinking becomes personally and socially acceptable and favored in the Irish culture. Measures targeting the whole population as well as specific at-risk groups are required. No single measure will be effective if taken in isolation. High prices and restriction of the availability of alcohol are the most effective measures, but this cannot be sustained long term without public support through information and advocacy. Measures targeting specific groups, especially young people, and specific settings, such as the workplace, along with accessible and effective treatment services will ensure a comprehensive policy.

CONCLUSION

A policy of awareness and understanding of the National Alcohol Policy and how it could be implemented in the respective areas of responsibility could create an effective network of support. Those who experience the problems related to substance abuse could, and must, establish an effective support network. These sectors that feel the effect of alcohol-related problems include health professionals such as doctors, nurses, and addiction counselors; the Gardai (police); social welfare officers; the judiciary; teachers; clergy; and the many voluntary agencies who provide support for those who have been affected by alcohol or other drug misuse.

The lack of alcohol and drug research in Ireland, with the exception of youth research, means that the Irish government relies too much on international research. The government needs clarification on important alcohol and drug-related issues, such as the economic, social, and psychological causes; the effects of substance-abuse consumption; the extent of drug dependence; and treatment effectiveness. There are also many unanswered questions in relation to the most effective treatment prevention models in different alcohol and drug cultures with a group and settings approach. This substance research must be improved to provide important measures for public health assessment and to allow for both effective and efficient use of resources, not only in Ireland, but around the world.

REFERENCES

Advertising Standards Authority of Ireland. (1995). *Code of advertising standards for Ireland*. Dublin: Author.

British Medical Association (1991). *The British Medical Association guide to medicine and drugs*. London: Darling Kindersley.

Conniffe, D. and McCoy, D. (2001). *Alcohol use in Ireland: Some economic and social implications*. Colorado Springs: International Academic Publishers.

Coopers and Lybrand (Eds.). (1994). *A guide to VAT in the EU: 1994 update*. Westport, CT: The Single Market Changes.

Department of Health and Children. (1996). *National Alcohol Policy*. Dublin: Author.

Dietler, M. (1994). "Our ancestors, the Gauls: Archaeology, ethnic nationalism, and the manipulation of Celtic identity in modern Europe." *American Anthropologist, 96* (3) 584–605.

Edwards, G. (1997). *Alcohol policy and the public good. Addiction, 92,* s73–s80.

Encarta Desk Encyclopedia (1998). *Ireland.* Microsoft Corporation on CD-ROM.

European Commission. (1993). *Inventory of taxes levied in the member states of the European communities* (15th ed.). Brussels: European Community.

Institute of Alcohol Studies (1997, March 26). *Ireland—Overview report on alcohol.* Cambridgeshire, England: Author.

Irish College of General Practitioners. (1991). *Submission to the advisory council on health promotion.* Dublin: Author.

McDonald, M. (1997). *Gender, drink and drugs.* New York: Oxford Press.

Morgan, M., and Grube, J.W. (1994). *Drinking among post-secondary school pupils.* Dublin: Economic and Social Research Institute.

National Roads Authority. (1994). *Road accident facts.* Dublin: Author.

Nic Gabhainn, S., & Kelleher, C.C. (1995). *Life skills for health promotion: The evaluation of the NWHB health promotion studies.* Galway: University College.

O'Kelley, M. (1999, December 15). Drug use common among students. *Ireland Examiner,* p. 1A.

Stack, P. (1996, February). "Kicking the habit." *Socialist Review.* (194). Retrieved on September 16, 2000 from the World Wide Web: http://www.lpi.org.uk.

9

MEXICO

Andrew Cherry and Irene Moreda

INTRODUCTION

Mexico is an important conduit in the illegal drug-trafficking pipeline that stretches from Colombia to Canada, and it has played that role for almost 100 years. Its identity as an illegal drug production and trafficking country began with the Harrison Narcotics Act of 1919, which made opium and heroin illegal in the United States. This law resulted in opium and heroin becoming contraband, and the more the authorities tried to restrict the trafficking of these drugs, the greater was the increase in the price of opium and heroin, and the greater were the profits for the drug traffickers.

Over the years, the illegal production and trafficking of drugs in Mexico have evolved to become an industry that is as sophisticated and complex as any of the other major industries in the world. The typical problem associated with illegal drug production and trafficking in Mexico during its early period was violence among the drug lords, the Mexican police, the Mexican army, the U.S. Border Patrol, the U.S. Coast Guard, and the U.S. Drug Enforcement Agency.

Alcohol addiction and the abuse of alcohol have been and continue to be common in Mexico; however, the number of alcoholics has remained about the same: roughly, 10 percent of the population have alcohol addiction problems. In the 1980s and 1990s, this changed when addiction to cocaine and heroin swept over the Mexican states located on the U.S. border. Increasingly, drugs that were being smuggled to the United States were also being sold to locals in these Mexican border towns and cities. As a result, by the year 2000, addiction and related substance-abuse problems, which people in the United States have struggled with for the last fifty years, were vanquishing the poor and and the middle class in many of Mexico's cities (Smith, 2000).

Apparently, the Mexican middlemen in the drug trade, who are often paid in drugs, began converting the drugs to cash by selling the drugs on the local Mexican market. Cocaine and heroin are the most popular hard drugs along the Mexican side of the border. For addicts on a budget, there is crystal methamphetamine. Made in household laboratories, it sells on the street in Tijuana for about $2 a hit (Zarembo, 2000).

This rapid increase in drug use and addiction has given rise to a growth industry in drug treatment and rehabilitation centers. Sadly, however, these drug-treatment centers are unregulated by the Mexican government. Typically, these centers are staffed by addicts who are themselves in recovery and who have little or no training. Consequently, the number of addicts who die during treatment has grown with the number of new drug treatment centers (Zarembo, 2000).

The role that Mexico plays on the world stage of drug abuse is unique among all other trafficking and drug-producing countries. How Mexico became a central player in the trafficking and production of illegal drugs, and how it is dealing with a new cohort of addicts, will help explain another facet of substance abuse around the world—the drug culture.

A Brief Profile of Mexico

Mexico, which includes a number of offshore islands, covers 758,452 square miles (1,964,382 square kilometers). The capital and largest city is Mexico City. The GDP was $335 billion (U.S.) in 1996, or about $3,725 (U.S.) per person.

The country of Mexico is made up of an elongated and elevated plateau that runs from north to the south of the country. This great plateau is flanked on both sides by two imposing mountain ranges. The mountain ranges are the Sierra Madre Occidental on the western coast and the Sierra Madre Oriental on the eastern coast. These mountain ranges fall off sharply to form narrow, low, flat coastal plains in the west and east. Mexico's longest river is the Rio Grande (called the Río Bravo del Norte in Mexico), which extends along the Mexican–U.S. border.

In general, the climate varies with elevation. On the humid, low coastal plains temperatures range from 16° to 49°C (60° to 120° F). At higher elevations average temperatures range from 15° to 21°C (59° to 70°F). Most of Mexico is relatively dry, although sections of southern Mexico receive significant precipitation.

Almost every known mineral is found in Mexico. There are large deposits of petroleum and natural gas. Forests cover 29 percent of the land, and 13 percent of Mexico is under cultivation. (*Encarta Desk Encyclopedia*, 1998).

The People of Mexico

In 1997 the population of Mexico was estimated to be 96,807,451. There are primarily three groups of people that make up the Mexican population: Mestizos, people of mixed European and Native American ancestry, who make up roughly 60 percent of the population; Native Americans, who constitute about 30 percent of the population; and, the group people of European descent, mostly Spanish. Approximately 76 percent of Mexico's people live in urban areas. Nearly 90 percent of the people in Mexico are Roman Catholic. The official language is Spanish. Education is free and compulsory for all children through age fifteen (Central Intelligence Agency, 2000).

Culture

Mexican culture is a complex blend of Native American, Spanish, and American traditions. The country has strong traditions of architecture, painting, writing, sculpture, handcrafts, and performing arts. Folk songs and dances are especially notable, including the *corrido*, a narrative folk ballad.

Mexico's economy reflects a shift from a primary-production economy, based on mining and agriculture, to a semi-industrialized economy. Mexican industries are among the most developed in Latin America. Mexican agriculture continues to supply most of the country's own foodstuffs. The primary crops are maize, sugarcane, sorghum, wheat, oranges, coffee, tomatoes, bananas, and potatoes. The most important fisheries lie off the coast of Baja California.

Most of Mexico's foreign trade is with the United States. Tourism, border trade, foreign investments, and the dollars sent back to Mexico by Mexican nationals working in the United States (typically sent to their families in Mexico) are significant sources of foreign exchange revenue (Central Intelligence Agency, 2000).

History

Mexico was the site of some of the earliest and most advanced civilizations in the Western Hemisphere. Mesoamerican civilizations included the Olmec, Maya, Toltec, and Aztec Indians. Based on reports from earlier European explorers, a small force under the command of Spanish explorer Hernán Cortés went to the Mexican territories hoping to find the elusive gold bonanza that was rumored to exist. Cortés quickly conquered the Aztecs, and Spain gained control of the region, which became known as New Spain.

Life in colonial Mexico was characterized by the exploitation of the Native Americans, the position and power of the Roman Catholic Church, and the existence of rigid social classes that supported people of pure European descent who held most of the powerful positions in New Spain.

By the beginning of the nineteenth century, resentment against Spanish rule, the inefficient government, and the occupation of Mexico by the French resulted in the Mexican war for independence. The Treaty of Córdoba in 1821, which marked Mexico's independence, was followed by many years of unstable and turbulent government. Revolt followed revolt until Antonio López de Santa Anna was elected president in 1833. During his reign a dispute with the United States, over the control of U.S. citizens moving into the Mexican region of Texas, ended in the Mexican War which lasted from 1846 to 1848. Mexico lost the war and signed the Treaty of Guadalupe Hidalgo in 1848, which fixed the Rio Grande as the boundary between Mexico and the United States. The war was politically and financially devastating for Mexico, and it was the beginning of another period of fierce struggle between Mexico's ruling classes and the liberal democrats (Suchlicki, 1996).

In the mid-1800s, Benito Pablo Juárez, a Native American, who modeled Mexico's constitution after the U.S. Constitution, idolized President Abraham Lincoln, even dressing in formal black suits and wearing a top hat like the one worn by Lincoln. At the urging of Juárez; a federal form of government, universal male suffrage, freedom of speech, and other civil liberties were written into the constitution of 1857. Conservative groups bitterly opposed the new constitution, which led to the War of the Reform in 1858, but by 1860 Juárez's forces had won the war. Elected president in 1861, Juárez suspended interest payments on foreign loans, which angered France, Britain, and Spain. In 1861 those countries sent a joint military expedition to Mexico. In 1863 Juárez and his cabinet fled, and a provisional conservative government proclaimed Mexico an empire and offered the crown to Maximilian, the archduke of Austria. In 1865 the occupying troops withdrew under pressure from the United States, and Juárez returned to power (Suchlicki, 1996).

In 1877 Porfirio Díaz, a former army general, was elected president. He ruled Mexico as a despot until he was forced to resign in 1911. National disorder continued until 1915, when a rebel leader, Venustiano Carranza, was internationally recognized as the lawful authority in Mexico. Another rebel leader, Francisco (Pancho) Villa, however, continued to disrupt the Mexican countryside until his army was defeated in 1920. Pancho Villa's army is the only army, other than the British army, to ever invade the United States. In 1941, as the United States was preparing for World War II, Mexico and the United States began a policy of cooperation that continues today (Suchlicki, 1996).

By the mid-1980s, the foreign debt had become an overwhelming burden, oil prices fell, and a devastating earthquake had plunged the country into a severe financial crisis. In 1992, to help the economy, President Carlos Salinas de Gortari (elected in 1988), U.S. President George H.W. Bush, and Prime Minister Brian Mulroney of Canada signed the North American

Free Trade Agreement (NAFTA), which created the largest free-trade zone in the world (Krauze, 1996).

In 1994, in the southern state of Chiapas, a group of Native Americans called the Zapatista National Liberation Army (known by the Spanish acronym EZLN) demanded reforms, including increased political power for indigenous Mexicans. This led to an armed conflict in which the economy was further strained by the unresolved situation in Chiapas (Suchlicki, 1996).

In July 1997 voters rejected the Partido Revolucionario Institucional (Institutional Revolutionary Party, or PRI), the largest and most important political party in Mexico. Opposition parties include the Partido de Acción Nacional (National Action Party, or PAN), a conservative, pro-Catholic group; and the Partido de la Revolución Democrática (Democratic Revolution Party, or PRD), a left-wing party (Krauze, 1996).

These political changes and the effect they will have on illegal production and trafficking has yet to be determined. However, if history is any indication of the future, it is likely that the production of illegal drugs and trafficking will be financially supporting the new political party in power. The supply of illegal drugs to the United States will not decrease, and if the United States demand does decline, the difference will be made up by the ever-growing number of Mexicans who are becoming addicted to illegal drugs which, in the past, were only sold in the United States (Krauze, 1996).

In the year 2000, some 14 percent of preteens in Mexico have used drugs. The national average was 5 percent. Drug use is even worse along the U.S.–Mexican border. Illegal drugs are cheaper and readily available in the border towns and cities (Avila, 2000).

VIGNETTE

In the Mexican drug culture, Tijuana, a city of 1.2 million people, is the home of Mexico's most violent cartel. More than 100 people were murdered in Tijuana in the first six months of the year 2000. This includes the killing of Tijuana's police chief in a barrage of automatic gunfire. Tijuana is also infamous for being the illegal-drug consumption capital of Mexico. In the 1990s, drug-rehabilitation centers, started by former drug addicts, began popping up like poppies in the fields. Starting with fewer than a dozen drug-treatment centers in 1994, there were over fifty treatment centers in Tijuana by the end of the year 2000. These centers are attempting to do what the Mexican government has not done—treat the exploding number of addicts in Tijuana. These centers, which are virtually unregulated, often rely on interventions that are outside of all accepted standard treatments. As such, the treatment interventions at best could be called very tough love. In far too many cases, the interventions have proved deadly (Zarembo, 2000). The following is the experience of one such recovering addict who opened a drug-rehabilitation center in Tijuana, and the treatment provided at his center.

In 1996, after more than ten years of shooting heroin, Hector M. checked himself into El Casa d'Oro, a rehabilitation center on the outskirts of Tijuana started and run by an ex-convict. In two weeks, he was given charge of six other addicts. Three months later, he was leading group-therapy sessions for sixty people a day and contemplating starting his own drug-rehabilitation center.

After staying clean for almost a year, Hector M. took his savings from his job as a taxi driver and rented a run-down house within sight of the border. The concrete walls of the house were crumbling and the outside was covered in faded graffiti. Even so, after cleaning out the trash and repairing the front door so it would close, Hector M. went around Tijuana telling the addicts he met that he was starting a rehabilitation center. His first client, a twenty-five-year-old woman from the United States, was addicted to heroin. To prevent her from running off during withdrawal, Hector M. tied her to a bed. She remained tied to the bed for more than five days.

After being open for about six months, Hector M. received a permit from the Mexican State Health Department to operate a drug-rehabilitation center. There were no minimum requirements; the application process consisted of sending in some identification and writing a letter explaining that he was opening a drug-rehabilitation center. Within a year of opening the center, fifty addicts were living in the house rented by Hector M. His fifty addicts shared mattresses that were laid on the floor during the night in the two largest rooms. They also shared the two bathrooms, one inside and one outside. Hector M. also lived in the house. Unlike his clients, he had a cellular telephone, a single bed in a small room at the back of the house, and a 1978 Honda.

A typical day at the center starts at 5 A.M. The ten guards—addicts who have been at the center for at least two weeks and have shown good behavior—remove the padlocks from the plywood bedroom doors. In the dirt yard behind the house, there are stacks of rusty bed frames, the top of a camper, and a weight bench with several barbells lying next to it. The residents brush their teeth and wash up in preparation for the day's events. Rap music blares from a boom box. One man shaves in front of a sliver of broken mirror using light from a light bulb hanging from a tree limb. Several other men sit together on an old sofa, sipping coffee in the early morning moonlight. By 5:45, with the mattresses leaning against the wall of the largest room, most of Hector's clients are packed into the room singing Christian hymns, bursting into coughing fits, listening to readings from the Narcotics Anonymous book, and sharing their stories of being down and out.

In the kitchen, thirty-three-year-old Marie A., one of the four women at the center, cooks tortillas for fifty. Electrical wires crisscross the ceiling and cupboards are filled with roaches and donated bread. Marie had been living on the streets of Tijuana selling herself to buy heroin to meet her uncontrollable drug habit. She had been in rehab before, but she had not been able to last more than two weeks. "Crystal, coke and crack have taken over their brains," she says. "One girl didn't even remember her name when she came in for treatment." By afternoon, the men are boiling pots of beans on an open fire in the driveway.

Nearby twenty-two-year-old Juan H. sits in a folding chair watching the activity. His job is to make sure nobody tries to run away. Like most of the addicts picked to be guards, he is large and intimidating. He wears a black T-shirt with a large marijuana leaf painted on the back; the name Roy is tattooed on his neck, in honor of a friend who was shot and killed in a gang fight over drug turf two years ago. His body is covered with stab wounds. Addicted to methamphetamine since he was thirteen years old, he had been in the center one month. It was the eighth time his mother had put him into a rehabilitation center. He says he does not want to return to his old ways, his old friends, and the gang he "ran with." Even so, after relapsing and being held in the garage (more like a jail) for several days, Juan ran away and returned to the streets after Hector let him out. Juan was soon arrested and imprisoned for assaulting a woman with a knife in an effort to steal money for methamphetamine.

In the back of the house, the small garage substitutes for a holding cell. Usually when a new client or old client is confined in the garage, several guards are assigned to monitor prisoners. The door of the garage is padlocked and the words "DETOX" are stenciled in Gothic letters above the door. A section of strong Hurricane fencing is nailed over the one window of the garage to keep the prisoners from escaping. Inside the garage, eleven men are neatly lined up on mattresses. Some appear to be asleep. The others watch television. One rather large fellow with a great mess of black hair and old and new track marks on his arms and neck rarely moves without groaning.

All new arrivals at Hector's center spend their first week locked in the garage/detox building. Hector might administer tranquilizers to those who experience the worst withdrawal symptoms to ease the effects of withdrawal. However, there are no doctors or nurses to determine the best medication, the appropriate dose, or when the medication should be given. Hector knows a doctor or nurse should be prescribing the medication, but sedatives are readily available without prescriptions in Mexico. Hector claims that, in more than a decade of addiction, he has learned more than most doctors know about dispensing sedatives and tranquilizers.

One prisoner is thirty-two-year-old Federico H. "They have no right to keep me here," he says through the bars. His parents had called Hector after finding drug paraphernalia in a trash can outside of their house. They had suspected their son was using drugs for some time. Federico was asleep when four of Hector's guards arrived at his parents' home. They went into his bedroom, handcuffed him, and carried him to a waiting car. After several days of protesting, Hector agreed to give Federico a drug test if his family would pay for it. With a guard watching him, Federico gave a urine sample. The next day the drug test came back clean and Federico was released. "It wasn't our decision to bring Federico here. It was his family. We're forced to believe them. All the family wants is to keep him from dying from drug addiction."

Rudolfo C. knew from experience how difficult it could be to force a person to accept drug treatment. Just two months earlier it had taken five men to catch him and lock him up in the detox room. He was given tranquilizers until he calmed down and went though withdrawal. Hector knows that kidnapping addicts and holding them against their will is against the law in Mexico, even if it is requested by the family. Nevertheless, kidnappings, tying addicts up so they cannot escape, addicts being given heavy psychotropic medication by people without formal training or the medical support if the patient overdoses on the medication, is still a common practice at these treatment centers.

At the center, around dusk, a dilapidated cab pulls up, and a male in his thirties gets out of the cab and hobbles unsteadily past the barking Dalmatian-mix, Freckles, to the front door of the center. Somebody had given him the address. Two other addicts lead him back to the garage. They take his belt and shoelaces—anything he could use to hurt himself—and he strips down to his underwear to make sure he is not hiding anything. His arms are covered in tattoos that hide some of the ugly tracks. He says he is ready to quit taking heroin. It was probably his best chance; however, after two difficult weeks of withdrawal, he leaves the center.

OVERVIEW OF SUBSTANCE ABUSE IN MEXICO AND BASIC DEMOGRAPHICS

Several social problems related to substance abuse have reached a critical level in Mexico. The growing number of drug addicts will continue to increase and spread across Mexico until prevention and public service campaigns are able to educate the Mexican people about the dangers of drug addiction and the violence that goes with it. The children who are living on the streets in the cities of Mexico are exploited by adults and the police; they use alcohol and illegal drugs; and the majority sniff glue or solvents they buy from dealers who specialize in selling glue to street children. Another major concern is the number of addicts who are dying in Mexican drug-treatment centers.

The Growing Number of Addicted

Mexican officials estimate that there are about 400,000 drug addicts, or 0.04 percent of Mexico's 100 million people. The numbers are relatively small when compared to the number of Mexicans who use legal drugs. Over 25 percent of the Mexicans are tobacco dependent, and 9.4 percent are addicted to alcohol. Illegal drug use, however, increased by more than 50 percent from 1988 to 1998. Specifically, 5.3 percent of the Mexican population acknowledged experimenting with illegal drugs at least once. This was up from 3.3 percent in 1988. In Tijuana, government pollsters recently registered a fivefold increase in drug use compared with a decade earlier. Women who are increasingly becoming addicted, in 1999 represented one in every thirteen drug addicts as compared to one in every twenty-three drug addicts in 1993 (Smith, 2000).

By comparison, in the United States, officials estimate that there are 3.6 million drug addicts (1.3 percent of the population), according to the White House Office of the U.S. National Drug Control Policy. Additionally, 10 percent of the U.S. population is addicted to alcohol—some 27.6 million people—according to the American Council on Alcoholism (Smith, 2000).

In the 1970s, few people in Tijuana knew anyone who had a drug problem. Since the mid-1990s, however, there is almost no family that has not experienced a drug problem at some level. And, there is not a Tijuana neighborhood that has not been affected by drugs and drug violence in some way.

The pattern of addiction in Mexico seems to be related to trafficking. Most Mexican drug dealers tend to become drug abusers and addicts. Completing the circle, all drug addicts will sell drugs to support their habit, if their addiction can be controlled long enough to complete a drug deal. Although accurate figures do not exist, in Mexico, long-term recovery rates after treatment for drug addiction are optimistically estimated to be somewhere between 20 to 30 percent (Smith, 2000).

Street Children and Glue

In Mexico City, like many other large cities in Mexico, and other Central and South American countries, there are large populations of street children. Bruce Harris, of the charity Casa Alianza, is working to change the life expectations of the street children in Mexico, Guatemala, and Honduras. The charity has a reputation of running excellent homes for street children. Harris has also pressed charges against police who have raped, assaulted, and even murdered street children. He brought a class action suit in the United States against the makers of Resistol glue, the most popular product for glue sniffers in Honduras where the child users are known as *Resistoleros* (Brennan, 1999).

Most street children in Mexico are very different from what one would expect. Not only are these children between ten and fifteen years old, as would be expected, but there are street children who are as young as three and four years old living as best they can, totally at the mercy of the streets. It is also not unusual to find newborn babies who are the children of street children. Nor is it unusual to find three generations of one family who have all been born in the streets of Mexico's cities (Klich, 1999).

Causes of Death in Mexican Treatment Centers

The Centros de Integracion Juvenil clinic in Tijuana is an example of drug rehabilitation centers in Mexico. The clinic is part of a nonprofit national chain that treats youth addictions. The Centros de Integración Juvenil provides ten weeks of treatment at a cost of up to $50 a week.

The problem with many of these Mexican drug-treatment centers is that too many addicts die while being treated at these centers. In 1998 and 1999, twenty addicts died who were being treated in Tijuana substance-abuse rehabilitation centers. The majority of those who die in drug treatment died from drug overdoses, hepatitis, heart attacks, HIV, and tuberculosis. A number of deaths, however, were caused by physical altercations with staff. In one case, two men from a drug-treatment center were jailed on homicide charges because of the death of a resident. The two staff members had taken thirty-five-year-old José Rodríguez N. to the Red Cross Hospital in Tijuana. By the time they arrived with Rodríguez, he was dead or near death. His body was bruised, several fingers were broken, and he had rope burns that indicated his wrists and ankles had been tied. The two men who were arrested were also patients at the same drug-treatment center where Rodríguez had died. The two men were involved because they were responsible for taking care of detox patients. They told prosecutors that Rodríguez was going through a rough withdrawal and that when he began bashing himself against a wall they tied him up. The head of the center did not know, for sure, what had happened. "We cannot make ourselves responsible for sick addicts. These types of things happen precisely because there are deficiencies. We cannot pay somebody to be there twenty-four hours a day" (Zarembo, 2000).

The head of the state human rights office, Antonio García Sánchez, says that he is limited to cases involving government agencies. Still, he receives about fifteen complaints a year of beatings and kidnappings by private drug-treatment centers. "They have proliferated out of control," he says. The majority of these private treatment centers take addicts by force. The families come looking for someone to save their addicted relatives. Because there are so few treatment options, "the authorities don't want to investigate too much." In private, some Mexican authorities make a grim argument for allowing the centers to continue operations. Yes, there have been problems, even deaths. The centers, nevertheless, take in people who have no other place to go—and who might otherwise die on the streets (Zarembo, 2000). In 2000, Mexican officials promised to establish regulations for drug treatment. The state legislature approved $640,000 to invest in the centers and began efforts to form a commission of government officials and rehabilitation center heads to set standards for the centers. The national health department is also preparing its own norms, which would outlaw locking up patients against their will, ban nonprofessionals from administering medicines, and require local health departments to have doctors on call who can be dispatched to the centers. Some centers would be shut down under the new rules (Zarembo, 2000).

HISTORY OF ALCOHOL AND DRUG ABUSE IN MEXICO

Drugs have been a part of Mexican culture for thousands of years. Drug trafficking also has a long history starting in Mexico before the turn of the twentieth century. Over the years, the farming and trafficking of illegal drugs have gone through many changes. These changes can help explain why illegal drugs became so plentiful in the second half of the twentieth century. These changes also reflect a political relationship between the United States and Mexico that has created a climate that gave birth to a drug subculture of illegal drug farmers, traffickers, and drug consumers on both sides of the border. These changes also help explain how this drug culture corrupted politicians and political institutions in Mexico and in the United States.

Alcohol has been used in Mexico for close to two thousand years. Alcohol was first made in Mexico from the sap of the blue agave plant (one of the American aloe plants), sometimes called the century plant. In fact, several of the agave plantations tended by the Aztec Indians in A.D. 1100 continue to be in production today. Most often today, however, the end product is tequila rather than the milky white liquor called pulque, a fermented drink similar to beer but not commercially available. It has an alcohol content of between 4 and 8 percent.

These native Americans also used drugs that had a similar effect to lysergic acid diethylamide (LSD), including peyote, mushrooms, and morning glory seeds. Peyote is a spineless cactus with a long, carrot-like root with a small crown or "button" that is psychoactive. The peyote button is first dried. Then the user holds the peyote in his or her mouth until it is soft. It is then swallowed without being chewed. Peyote was used for thousands of years in religious ceremonies by the Aztecs, other Mexicans, and North American Indian tribes. Based on archaeological finds, there also appears to have been a mushroom religious cult in Guatemala over 3,500 years ago. Morning glory seeds were also being used by the natives to the extent that they were referred to as the "diabolic seed" by ecclesiastical authorities in the 1500s.

Although rare, mushrooms and peyote continue to be used by the Central American and North American Indians in traditional religious ceremonies (Brecher, 1972).

Among the people of Mexico, as in all countries of the world in the nineteenth century and the beginning of the twentieth century, drugs such as marijuana, opiates, and cocaine were commonly used, and opiates were widely used in medication. The most commonly abused opiate was laudanum, a mix of alcohol and opium. The most popular opium derivatives were morphine and heroin. Cocaine, coca wines, and marijuana cigarettes were prescribed by doctors and easily obtained in pharmacies. During this period, the government's interest in these drugs was to ensure the quality of these products to protect the buyers. Addicts were considered to be "sick" people, not criminals. A poppy-growing culture developed in Mexico in the 1880s in the northwestern state of Sinaloa. Although it is not well documented, apparently the Chinese brought the poppy seeds to Sinaloa, Mexico, and much of the opium produced there was sold to the Chinese living on the West Coast of the United States. Mexico attempted to control laudanum, opium, and marijuana for nonmedical use between 1870 and the 1900s with little success (Astorga, 1999).

This situation changed in the early 1900s. The Shanghai Conference in 1909, orchestrated by the United States, called for opium controls around the world. It was the beginning of U.S. "drug diplomacy," a policy that continues to influence the regulation of drugs internationally. At the Shanghai Conference, U.S. politicians convinced or coerced other countries to accept opium control. The Harrison Narcotics Act was passed by the U.S. Congress in 1914 and signed into law by President Woodrow Wilson in 1916. This law was presented as a model for other countries to follow. The Harrison Act was designed to control opium production, sales, and consumption in the United States.

In 1917 a Mexican congressman, Dr. José María Rodríguez, proposed an amendment that gave powers to the Mexican congress to dictate laws on citizenship, naturalization, colonization, emigration and immigration, and general health in the country. Among the reasons for the amendment was concern about alcoholism and the "selling of substances that poison the individual and degenerate the [Mexican] race." He named opium, morphine, ether, cocaine, and marijuana. The purpose was to interrupt their "immoderate or non-medical use." According to him, mortality had increased because of the lack of official control of those drugs (Astorga, 1999).

In the years immediately following the passage of the Harrison Act (1916 to the mid-1920s), most of the illicit opium drug trade went through Mexicali and Tijuana, in Baja California. The cultivation and commercialization of marijuana were prohibited in Mexico in 1920; poppy cultivation and opium production, in 1926. According to Mexican officials, the argument that persuaded Mexican lawmakers to pass the law was "race degeneration" (Astorga, 1999).

During this period, the number of Mexicans addicted to opium, or other drugs, was small. Drug use and abuse in Mexico were not widespread, and the number of people who were addicted was far less than those addicted in the United States. Marijuana was generally used by Mexican soldiers, criminals, and poor people. Opium smoking was confined to Chinese minorities; and morphine, heroin, and cocaine were used by degenerate artists, middle-class people, and the bourgeoisie. The drug traffickers' main business was north of the Mexican border, and did not impact the average Mexican.

Drug Trafficking in Sinaloa

Sinaloa is a long, narrow state in northwestern Mexico which runs north and south along Mexico's western coast. Mexico's most important fishery state, it is also the second leading producer of vegetables and cereals in Mexico. In the mountains farmers have been growing marijuana for hundreds of years and opium poppies for the last 150 years. As such, Sinaloa has a special place in the history of illegal drugs and trafficking in Mexico. In the 1930s, the people living in Sinaloa even coined the word *gomeros* to describe the opium traffickers in that Mexican state. In the saloons frequented by these *gomeros*, alcohol, music, and pistols were a deadly combination. The reasons for the shootings were not always related to drug affairs, but some traffickers began to use the saloons and the neighborhoods in which they lived as battlefields. For that reason, in the 1950s, the press in Culiacán (the capital of Sinaloa) named the city "a new Chicago with gangsters in sandals." The illegal drug business had grown up in Sinaloa, and so had the violence associated with it (Astorga, 1999).

The Volstead Act of 1919

The one event that contributed the most to the development of Mexico as a drug-trafficking country was the Volstead Act which, like the Harrison Narcotics Act, became law in the United States in 1919. The Volstead Act prohibited the production, sale, and consumption of alcohol in the United States. The Harrison Act prohibited the production, sale, and consumption of opium products in the United States. In Mexico, however, the production, sale, and consumption of alcohol and opium were legal. The difference in the laws of the two countries created the conditions for developing a sophisticated alcohol- and drug-trafficking organization. There was a great deal of money to be made by smuggling illegal alcohol into the United States. The Mexican traffickers already had the routes and retail contacts, including political protection. When the Volstead Act became law, the informal smuggling operations quickly went into the business of rum running. (Astorga, 1999).

Mexican drug traffickers were not the only ones who changed their business practices with the passage of the Volstead Act. In the United States, in the first six months after the Volstead Act became law, more than 15,000 physicians and 57,000 druggists and drug manufacturers applied for licenses to prescribe and sell alcohol. By 1928 U.S. physicians were making an estimated $40 million per year by writing prescriptions that had alcohol as the main ingredient (McWilliams, 1990).

The Marijuana Tax Act

Albeit there were some marijuana users in the United States in the 1930s, their numbers were small. Marijuana traffickers from Mexico typically sold their marijuana to Mexican nationals who had migrated to the United States to work in the fields and factories in California and Texas. These early Mexican traffickers were poorly organized. Most of the marijuana smuggled into the United States was grown and smuggled by people living in Sinaloa and other Mexican states along the border. The same farmers who grew marijuana also cultivated poppies, and the opium was smuggled to the Chinese in California. The trafficking routes and families who had traditionally smuggled marijuana and opium began smuggling alcohol as well (McWilliams, 1990).

After the Harrison Narcotics and Volstead acts became law in 1919, the next major event in Mexico's experience with U.S. drug laws was orchestrated by Harry J. Anslinger, chief of the Bureau of Narcotic Drugs. He focused on marijuana as one of the last drugs being used in the United States that was not outlawed by the earlier Harrison Act. After creating mass hysteria about the threat of marijuana, the Marijuana Tax Act was approved in 1937 (McWilliams, 1990).

The Development of the Narco-Economy in Mexico

In the 1960s, the demand by students and U.S. soldiers for marijuana exploded. In 1966 Mexican officials reported the destruction, in forty-five days, of 3,000 tons of marijuana in two marijuana-growing states: Chihuahua and Sinaloa. In 1968 Look magazine estimated the marijuana being smuggled from Mexico into the United States at around 3.5 to 5 tons per week. In 1969 President Richard Nixon launched Operation Intercept to stop the inflow of marijuana. This was the beginning of a new era of drug policies in the United States (McWilliams, 1990).

Since the 1960s, the U.S. demand for marijuana, heroin, and cocaine has brought enormous wealth to a few drug traffickers in Mexico. However, the politicians and the banking centers of Mexico have derived even greater profits from the narco-industry. Officials estimated the Mexican traffickers' profits in 1994 to be $30 billion—a sum that is four times the value of the national oil revenues. Thirty billion dollars was 7.1% of the Mexican GNP in 1994. International authorities estimated that somewhere between $8 and 30 billion narco-dollars were circulating in Mexican banks in 1996. These profits were so high that most could not resist and if they did, they were often killed. Additionally, there is strong evidence in the form of reports and studies to suggest that law enforcement was a political tool. Although through the years a few major traffickers and politicians have been arrested and jailed, these events were more the result of one drug lord's taking over the other's business than it was a political or law enforcement operation (McWilliams, 1990).

The drug problem that the people of Mexico share with their pre-Colombian brothers and sisters is alcohol abuse and addiction. Prior to the arrival of the Europeans, the only drug that caused problems for individuals, families, and society was alcohol in the form of pulque. The other drugs that are now illegal were used until recently without the user's suffering from dependence or addiction. However, since the 1980s, addiction to cocaine and heroin has rapidly increased following the trend in the United States (Suchlicki, 1996).

SUBSTANCE ABUSE IN MEXICO TODAY

In the early 1990s, when drug addiction was rapidly spreading along the Mexico–U.S. border, professionals in the field of addiction were concerned that it would reach down into the heartland of Mexico, and it did. By 1997 cocaine addiction had become a serious problem in the slums of Mexico City. Drug dealers invaded working-class neighborhoods. Gangs were armed and shootings were common. Children were no longer safe when playing outside. Some of the dealers were selling drugs in the schools. Addiction began to cause family breakups, and violence and crime increased (Riley, 2000).

Some analysts suggest that U.S. drug policy may have inadvertently contributed to the upsurge in drug use in Mexico. By pushing Mexico to increase its fight against drugs, the informal agreement between the illegal drug cartels and the Mexican government began to fall apart. The government had informally agreed that they would not come down too hard on the drug traffickers, and traffickers would not put drugs on the streets of the cities in Mexico (Riley, 2000).

Political Views and Public Policies

By the late 1930s, marijuana was being produced by the ton in Puebla, Guerrero, and Tlaxcala. Of the alleged owners of the farms, several who lived in Mexico City were suspected of being protected by high-ranking members of the anti-narcotics police. Political protection went unchecked until after World War II. The first major scandal related to political corruption broke in 1947 when General Pablo Macías Valenzuela, the ex-secretary of war and navy (national defense) and governor of the state of Sinaloa (1945–1950), was suspected of leading a drug-trafficking ring or protecting opium traffickers. This was only the first of many similar political scandals. Since the beginning of drug smuggling, the best-known drug traffickers in Mexico were identified with Mexican high-ranking politicians (Astorga, 1999).

The Mexican government spent $170 million in 1999 on drug interdiction, much of which went to acquire new ships, helicopters, and satellite tracking equipment—all of no use in fighting street drugs (Riley, 2000).

Social Views, Customs, and Practices

If there is any doubt that a highly developed drug culture exists in Mexico, all one has to do is listen to a popular Mexican radio station. Mexican pop songs, known as *corridos*, glorify the country's "cocaine cowboys," glorifying their riches and ignoring the dark side of illegal drug trafficking—violence, addiction, and death or imprisonment. With titles such as "The King of Drugs" and "A Trafficker's Empire," the *corridos* have made the trafficker, with his automatic weapons, his silver-studded belts and boots, and his cowboy hat, the role model for Mexican youths seeking to escape poverty (Astorga, 1999).

Yet, it is not just the poor Mexican youth and the drug dealers who have been entrapped by drug abuse. Much of the country's wealth and violence are directly related to Mexico's narco-economy and drug-trafficking culture. Mexico City has become one of the most dangerous cities in the world. Crime has escalated rapidly since Mexico's 1994 economic collapse and is increasing about 35 percent a year (Diebel, 1999).

There has also been a "democratization" of crime in Mexico. People who used to feel safe, such as celebrities, business people, and other wealthy residents, are the new preferred targets. By the year 2000, narco-crime had spread out from the poor neighborhoods and into suburban communities. It also claimed the entertainment and law enforcement sector of Mexico. Alejandro Gertz, Mexico City's police chief in 1999, had to fire most of the city's police superintendents and division chiefs. Corruption was so pervasive that Gertz sent a letter to Mexico City's 36,000 uniformed police officers, begging them to turn in their own bosses. "If any of you suffer pressure or orders from your bosses to extort people, I want you to call my office right away," Gertz wrote in the open letter sent to all precincts. Consequently, Gertz arrested and charged forty-four top-ranking police officers with crimes ranging from rape and murder to corruption. He also offered bonuses to police officers (about $30) who made an arrest in connection with a violent crime. Although some in Mexico City demanded Gertz fire the entire police force and start over with a new police force, others pointed out that when thousands of police officers were fired in the past, the city ended up with thousands of armed, unemployed cops on the street, many of whom became criminals themselves (Diebel, 1999).

THE FUTURE OF SUBSTANCE ABUSE IN MEXICO

The substance-abuse problem seen now in the streets of Mexican cities will increase in the twenty-first century. When the demand for illegal drugs leveled off in the United States in the late 1990s, more and cheaper illegal drugs became available in Mexico. As the number of addicts increase and treatment is not available or is ineffective, the number of lives and families destroyed by substance abuse will continue to grow in Mexico. Prevention and public service campaigns must be developed to counter the drug culture among the young people of Mexico, especially the poor youth who have few or no options to a better life, unless they succeed in the illegal drug trade. When many of these teenagers dream of the future, they know the only realistic option they have, if they wish to taste the fruits of the world, is to become a successful trafficker in drugs or people between Mexico and the United States. Although all other options are closed to the majority of Mexico's poor youth, there is always an opening for teenage drug dealers.

Political corruption on both sides of the Mexican–U.S. border provides a fairly safe environment for smuggling illegal drugs into the United States. Even with the losses of drug shipments as reported in the world press, the profits are enormous for the traffickers and corrupt politicians. On the world market, only arms sales generate more commerce than illegal drugs. Money laundering on an international scale supports these illegal operations. However, without a way of laundering the money to hide the fact that the money was earned by selling illegal drugs, neither politicians nor traffickers would have access to such enormous wealth. A billion dollars in cash is a lot of money, but if it cannot be converted into certificates of deposit, the cash is of little good, especially when every transaction over $10,000 has to be reported to the authorities.

The children living on the streets of Mexico's cities will continue to be a serious problem. Their lives will be cut short by violence and drug abuse. Too often, teenage girls who grew up on the streets are giving birth and raising a second generation of children in the streets of Mexican cities. These children live their lives on the streets because of failed social policies that need attention. More must be done to protect and rehabilitate street children, and to prevent others from becoming street children.

Proposed Solutions and Strategies

Beginning in the year 2000, the Mexican National Health Department began preparing its own policy and procedures for regulating Mexican drug-treatment centers. One plan is to require local health departments to have doctors on call who can be dispatched to the centers if a resident were medically compromised (Zarembo, 2000). This is a good start, but regulations must be developed and enforced so that, at a minimum, they provide for legal penalties for centers that lock up patients against their will. The regulations must require that only medical professionals prescribe and administer medicines. Furthermore, after providing training to drug-treatment personnel, centers that continue to use harsh and abusive handling as an intervention for drug use or as a part of detoxification procedure should be closed.

Prevention programs such as Youth Day on the Mexico–United States Border are notable attempts to prevent an increase in drug use and addiction among Mexico's youth. This program was promoted by concerned community leaders who wanted to move from concern to action in an effort to prevent the problem of drug use from growing among the young (Avila, 2000).

The government of the Republic of Mexico began putting more resources into prevention and drug-treatment programs in the late 1990s. Even so, the budget is small compared to the budget for the interdiction and eradication of illegal drug crops (Avila, 2000). One approach to deal with the growing drug use and addiction problems in Mexico would be for the Mexican government to negotiate a provision in the next treaty in the U.S. drug war to provide a percentage of the money given to Mexico for military operations to eradicate drug crops and to provide drug treatment to the victims of the drug war, the addicts.

The money-laundering problem must deal with the source of corruption. The large sums of money will continue to corrupt Mexico's politicians and thus the Mexican political, governmental, and legal institutions. However, this cannot be accomplished at the national level. It can work only if there is nowhere in the world drug lords can turn their mountains of cash into legitimate certificates of deposits.

The United States and Canada must also take responsibility for the role Mexico plays in the international drug culture. By dominating all legal markets and aggressively preventing the development of legal products that could be manufactured or grown in Mexico, these juggernaut nations have left Mexico and other countries in the Caribbean and Central and South America with no other source of income. If marijuana, cocaine, and heroin were legalized today, their prices would plummet and the narco-economy would collapse, as would the economies of most of the world's developing countries. Before the narco-economy is destroyed, another way for the drug producers (thousands of small farmers and intermediaries) to earn a living for their families must be developed.

CONCLUSION

There are many more alcoholics in Mexico than drug addicts. Even so, the number of drug addicts has been growing since the mid-1990s. The numbers show no sign of declining or even leveling off. Yet, the increasing number of drug addicts is only one of the faces of substance abuse devastating Mexico. Its political, legal, and legitimate business communities have been badly compromised by the enormous wealth involved in the trafficking of illegal drugs.

This is a problem that Mexico cannot solve in isolation. The substance-abuse problem is a worldwide problem. It is a problem because of the inclination of most humans to use psychoactive substances and the propensity for about 10 percent of the human population to become addicted to a psychoactive agent. The number of humans who become addicted will not change if these psychoactive drugs are legal or illegal. The profits and enormous wealth involved in the trafficking of illegal drugs is a dynamic condition. This condition can be changed. The profits going to the drug lords, criminals who also have legitimate business, and corrupt politicians could be stopped by legalizing the commerce in psychoactive drugs. Mexico has a history of growing and selling both marijuana and opium as legal crops. They could resume that role with little effort.

REFERENCES

Astorga, L. (1999). *Drug trafficking in Mexico: A first general assessment.* Discussion Paper no. 36. Paris: UNESCO. Downloaded on September 20, 2000, from the World Wide Web: http://www.unesco.org/

Avila, J.A.O. (2000). *Severe addiction rates among the inhabitants of our northern border.* Worldsources Online, Inc. Downloaded on September 20, 2000, from the World Wide Web: http://www.elibrary.com.

Brecher, E.M. (1972). *Licit and illicit drugs.* Boston: Little Brown.

Brennan, D. (1999, September 14). Law: What they need is a lawyer. *The Independent* (London), p. 14.

Central Intelligence Agency. (2000). *The world factbook: Mexico.* Washington, D.C.: prepared by the Central Intelligence Agency for the use of U.S. government officials. Retrieved on September 26, 2000, from the World Wide Web: http://www.odci.gov/cia/publications/factbook/geos/fr.html

Diebel, L. (1999, June 20). Killing of popular TV host triggers Mexican scandal. *Toronto Star,* p. 1A.

Encarta Desk Encyclopedia (1998). Microsoft Corporation on CD-ROM.

Klich, K. (1999, March 20). Mean streets: The streets of Mexico City are home to thousands of destitute children whose lives are marred by drug addiction, sickness, and abuse by the police. *The Independent* (London), pp. 1, 11–14.

Krauze, E. (1996). *Mexico: Biography of power*. New York: HarperCollins.

McWilliams, J.C. (1990). *The Protectors. Harry J. Anslinger and the Federal Bureau of Narcotics, 1930–1962*. Newark: University of Delaware Press.

Riley, M. (2000, February 29). Drug problems flow back south of the border: Mexico reports increase in cocaine addiction cases. *Houston Chronicle*, p. A1.

Smith, E.B. (2000, September 12). Mexico's drug trade taking down its citizens: Abuse problems now touching all walks of life. *USA Today*, p. 22A.

Suchlicki, J. (1996). *Mexico: From Montezuma to NAFTA, Chiapas, and beyond*. Dulles, VA: Brassey's.

Zarembo, A. (2000, March 20). Tough love in Tijuana. *Newsweek*, p. 26. Downloaded on September 20, 2000, from the World Wide Web: http://www.elibrary.com.

10

THE NETHERLANDS

Andrew Cherry

INTRODUCTION

The Netherlands, known unofficially as Holland, is an important country to study when trying to understand substance abuse. It is important because the Netherlands is the only developed country that has gone down a different road in its effort to deal with a continuing and persistent worldwide drug problem and its effect on people around the world, in particular, its effect on young people. In the early 1970s, a shopping cart full of different and intriguing drugs became available to the public. Teenagers in most developed countries, who could not legally purchase alcoholic beverages, regarded these drugs as an alternative. Even more fascinating, the new drugs provided a variety of intoxicating experiences that were different from being drunk on alcohol. Most older adults and political leaders around the world regarded this loss of control over youthful behavior dangerous to young people. The government dusted off the laws passed between 1919 and 1932, which were designed to control heroin, cocaine, and marijuana, and began to enforce these laws vigorously, particularly against the youth. In turn, college youth began developing synthetic drugs that were not illegal and in many cases had never been heard of before. As fast as students designed new synthetic recreational drugs, and the synthetics hit the streets, legislators outlawed them.

In the early 1970s, the Dutch used the prohibition model to guide public policy in drug control, but by the mid-1970s, it was clear to most Dutch that prohibition was not reducing the drug problem. It was also clear that, in this small country, the prohibition approach was resulting in the flooding of the prisons and jails, not with criminals, but with the sons and daughters of families from all levels of society—whose only crime was possessing a controlled substance. Because Holland is a small, tightly knit community with a tradition of tolerance in religion and other matters, the Dutch realized that the laws punishing youthful drug users were far more harmful than the drugs being used by the teenagers. While other countries were building more prisons to house the drug users, arming their police for combat, and giving the authorities unprecedented authority of search and seizure in peacetime, Holland tried a different approach.

Dutch politicians chose to tackle the drug problem by legalizing soft drugs and reducing the penalty for using other drugs. At the same time, the government pledged to fight trafficking of all drugs, particularly trafficking in hard drugs, such as heroin and cocaine, and synthetic drugs, including methamphetamines (Cohen, 1996).

The Dutch Example

"Look at the Dutch example!" This has become the call to arms for both those opposed to liberalizing drug laws and those who support liberalizing drug laws. In 1979 the Dutch parliament set Holland's drug policy on a course of its own—one markedly different from that of the rest of world, one not dictated by U.S. drug policy or by U.S. drug diplomacy. The Dutch legislators legalized the public sale of cannabis products (under certain conditions) in their now famous (or infamous) coffee shops. They also wrote and adopted legislation that takes a more lenient approach toward all forms of drug use and abuse based on a philosophy of "harm reduction" (Collins, 1999).

In this chapter, the consequences of that policy are examined in terms of the impact on Dutch society and the impact on the number of addicts in the Netherlands. This chapter also examines the questions about the effect of their policies on drug use and the incidence of addiction in Holland. Dutch drug policies are also examined in terms of their impact on various neighbors, including France, Belgium, Germany, and the United Kingdom. Do the results justify considering the Dutch drug policy an alternative to the prohibition model?

In the 1970s, advocates of Holland's harm-reduction policy argued that providing soft-drug users with a shopping outlet in which to buy their drugs would keep them from falling prey to drug pushers and the criminal element involved in drug trafficking. Those Dutch who wished to experiment or use soft drugs would have a source that would not require them to interact with hard-drug users and sellers. It was predicted that petty crime would fall and that fewer young people would use and become addicted to hard drugs. Were the predictions correct? In 1997 the results of this twenty-year experience with the Dutch harm-reduction model were evaluated (Netherlands Ministry of Health, Welfare and Sports 1999a).

The 1997 progress report on hard-drug use in the Netherlands, conducted by the government-financed Trimbos Institute, estimated the number of heroin addicts in Holland to be 25,000 individuals. The estimated number was based on the number of heroin addicts who actually came into contact in one way or another with the nation's social or justice departments. Critics say the real figure is closer to 35,000, although they offer no hard data to support their estimated numbers.

Drug addiction has remained more or less stable since 1980, and it is lower than in most other European countries. Addiction to soft drugs (cannabis products: hash, hash oil, and the leaf and buds) has been relatively rare over the last twenty years. In 1997 there were about 2,500 addicts, or 0.0037 percent of the population of cannabis users. There is 1 addicted cannabis user for every 270 users of cannabis. About 25,000 people are addicted to hard drugs. Ecstasy (XTC) was also being widely abused at the beginning of the twenty-first century, particularly at teenage parties and at nightclubs that attract young people. The number of hard-drug-related deaths due to accidental and other narcotic poisoning fluctuates at around 60 per year; the death rate among the 350,000 Dutch who use alcohol is 1,600 each year. There were 0.45 percent deaths annually among alcohol users and 0.15 percent deaths among heroin or narcotics users. Although the Netherlands is known for its lax hard-drug laws, in terms of harm, for every 1 person that dies from hard drugs, 26 people die from alcohol-related disorders (Spuit and van Laar, 1997).

Referring to Holland's drug policies, enacted first in 1979, Dr. Ernest Bunning of the Netherlands Public Health Ministry said, in a 1999 interview,

I would not be proud if we were to be seen by our neighbors as a narco-state. . . . We don't want people to come here just to get stoned and gawk at the girls in the windows [prostitutes regulated by law who stand in the window of the "shops" to advertise their availability]. . . . We have a culture and a history of which we are proud. . . . With drugs we are in the realm of theory. There is no simple solution to the drug problem. No one nation, not the U.S., not England, has the answer. But our solution in Holland is not ideal either. (Collins, 1999, p. 82).

A Brief Profile of The Netherlands

The Netherlands is a country in northwestern Europe, west of Germany and north of Belgium. The Netherlands Antilles and Aruba, islands in the Caribbean Sea, are also considered part of the Netherlands. The European mainland of the Netherlands has a total area of 16,033 square miles (41,526 square kilometers). The capital and largest city is Amsterdam (Netherlands Board of Tourism, 2000).

Almost everyone has heard the parable of the little Dutch boy who stuck his finger in a hole of a dike that had sprung a leak. The Netherlands, a low-lying country on the North Sea of the Atlantic coast, yearly experiences severe storms. Almost half of the country is below sea level. The coastline extends out into the Atlantic as a series of sand dunes. Behind the dunes the land that is below sea level is protected from flooding by a system of dikes, dams, and locks. It is kept dry by continuous mechanical pumping. The country's largest lake, the IJsselmeer, is an artificial lake that was created as part of a continuing project to reclaim land from the sea. Major rivers include the Rhine, the Maas, and the Schelde. As land is scarce and fully utilized, there are few areas of forest and no wilderness areas. The forests that are preserved are carefully managed. Grasslands and meadows provide habitats for rabbits, but larger wildlife have long since died out (*Encarta Desk Encyclopedia*, 1998).

The People of Holland

The Netherlands is one of the world's most densely populated countries with a population of 15,649,729 (1997 estimate). Nearly 90 percent of the people live in urban areas. Roman Catholics constitute about 33 percent of the population and Protestants, 23 percent. Thirty-nine percent of the Dutch do not claim church membership. Public schools account for about a third of the schools in Holland; the remainder of schools are private schools operated by religious groups. Both public and private schools receive public financing. School attendance is compulsory from ages five to sixteen (*Encarta Desk Encyclopedia*, 1998).

After World War II, Rotterdam became a leading center for refining petroleum, and in recent decades the Netherlands has become the world's fifth largest exporter of natural gas. The Dutch currency is the guilder (1.70 guilders equaled U.S.$1 in 1996). In 1997 the gross domestic product (GDP) of the Netherlands was $360.3 billion, or $24,000 per individual. This is a sizable GDP per person. The GDP in the United States in 1998 was $8.40 trillion, or about $20,000 per person (Netherlands Board of Tourism, 2000).

Government

The Netherlands government is a constitutional monarchy (the monarchy has no political power) with a parliamentary system of government. The ceremonial head of state is the monarch. The prime minister is responsible to the States-General, which consists of a 75-member First Chamber, elected to four-year terms by the provincial legislatures, and a 150-member Second Chamber, popularly elected to terms of up to four years (*Encarta Desk En-*

cyclopedia, 1998). Interestingly, although Amsterdam is the capital of the Netherlands, the government holds its meetings in The Hague.

Historical Holland

The Netherlands first appeared in history when the Romans conquered the Germanic and Celtic tribes inhabiting the area in the first century B.C. After several thousand years of being taken over by kings and emperors, in 1555 Hapsburg Emperor Charles V gave the Netherlands to his son, Philip II, the emperor of Spain. In part because of the repressive policies of Philip II and the dissatisfaction with the Roman Catholic Church, in 1566 anti-Catholic riots spread across Holland. Philip sent Spanish troops to quell the riots, which resulted in open revolt. William I, Prince of Orange, led the Dutch in the capture of most of the northern territory. In 1579 the Union of Utrecht, an alliance of all northern and some southern territories, was formed. The provinces that joined the union became the Netherlands; those territories that did not join became Belgium. In 1581 the Union of Utrecht proclaimed independence from Spain. After numerous wars and campaigns, the Spanish recognized the sovereignty of the Dutch Republic in 1648.

Starting in the early 1600s vessels sailing from Amsterdam to Indonesia developed lucrative Dutch trading stations throughout the world. By the mid-1600s, the Netherlands was the foremost commercial and maritime power in Europe (Newton, 1978).

During this period of expansionism, the Dutch and the English came into conflict over these trade routes. Two Anglo-Dutch Wars were waged during the 1650s and 1660s. Other wars were waged against France. In 1810 Napoléon Bonaparte incorporated the Low Countries of Holland into the French empire. After the fall of Napoléon, the kingdom of the Netherlands was restored. The second half of the nineteenth century witnessed a liberalization of the Dutch government. Suffrage was gradually extended, and agitation for social reform increased. During World War II (1939–1945), the Netherlands was occupied by the Germans and suffered heavy destruction. The years following the war were marked by intensive efforts to rebuild the country and regain their lost colonies (Newton, 1978).

The Dutch are a prosperous people, conservative by nature, who place a high value on an individual's right to take certain risks that are not a nuisance to the community at large. This philosophy is the result of a history of Dutch struggles to acquire and maintain individual and national freedom. When faced with a drug problem spiraling out of control and faced with the choice of building more prisons or letting the drug users go free, the Dutch decriminalized the sale of cannabis and decriminalized the use of all drugs. The change in drug laws reduced the number of people in Dutch prisons and stopped the arrests and prosecution of users, which in turn released more resources for prosecution of criminal trafficking groups, for drug-prevention programs, and for increasing the availability of treatment (Netherlands Ministry of Health, Welfare and Sports, 1997).

VIGNETTE

Near Rotterdam's modern and clean Marconiplein subway station there is a line of dilapidated brick buildings; at least half of them are uninhabited and boarded up. This is Rhijnvis Feithstraat in Spangen. Years ago, it was a respectable lower-class neighborhood inhabited by families struggling to make ends meet. By the late 1990s, most of the residents along the street were drug dealers, who openly sold heroin, cocaine, crack, and Ecstasy. The police estimate that there are 200 such houses operating in Rotterdam at any given time. The dealers sublet the buildings from people who subleased the buildings from another tenant. This arrangement hides the identity of the building's owner. They rent out rooms for about 200 guilders (approximately U.S.$120) a day. The people who sublease the rooms sell high-grade heroin, amphetamines, cocaine, crack, Ecstasy, and any other drug for which there is a market. Heroin sells for about 80 guilders (U.S.$50) a gram; this is about a third of what it costs in other EU countries. The Dutch police know where these houses are located; however, the police policy in most of Rotterdam, as in most other Dutch cities, is to tolerate the drug houses at least until neighbors complain. This has resulted in some interesting relationships between the drug dealers and their neighbors. The golden rule among dealers is, "Don't bother the neighbors, and the police won't bother us." When neighbors need a hand with a community project, the dealers pitch in and help. When a neighbor has a financial crisis, the dealers organize a charity drive.

In Rotterdam, another approach has been used to reduce harm to hard-drug addicts. The approach was designed and run by a middle-aged woman named Nora Storm, the president of the city's drug addicts' trade union, the Junkiebund. A number of houses were set up with rooms for addicts. Drug dealers specifically assigned to the addict houses sold the addicts their daily drug fix. The addicts paid for their drugs by cleaning the Rotterdam city streets for 50 guilders a day (about U.S.$25), enough money to buy a day's supply of their drugs. The hope was that, by giving addicts a stable environment and a normal work routine, some of the addicts would eventually kick the habit. The police knew which houses Storm ran and ignored the drug sales being made at the houses. The number of addicts in her program who have gone into treatment and kicked the habit is unknown. Even so, it demonstrates the willingness of the Dutch to try different approaches to the prevention and treatment of drug use, abuse, and addiction.

Table 10.1
Drug Deaths per Year in the Netherlands: The Number of Drug Users and
Drugs Causing Deaths

	Cannabis	Heroin and Narcotics	Alcohol	Tobacco
Number of Users	675,000	40,000	350,000	5,000,000
Percentage of Population	4%	0.026%	2%	33%
Number of Deaths	0	60	1,600	17,600
Percentage of Population	0%	0.0015%	0.0046%	0.0035%

Source: Dufour, van der Haar, and van der Hoeven, 1996.

OVERVIEW OF SOCIAL ISSUE AND BASIC DEMOGRAPHICS

In order to understand the Dutch approach to the drug problem, it is useful to remember that the Netherlands is one of the most densely populated, urbanized countries in the world. It has a population of 15.5 million and occupies an area of no more than 16,033 square miles. The Dutch firmly believe in the freedom of the individual, with the government playing no more than a background role in religious or moral issues. A cherished feature of Dutch society is the free and open discussion of such issues. A high value is attached to the well-being of society as a whole. The Netherlands has an extensive social security system, and everyone has access to health care and education. These social proclivities coalesced in a harm-reduction philosophy and social interventions to deal with the overwhelming drug problem faced by the Dutch as well as developed nations in the 1960s (Cohen, 1996).

Consequently, drug addiction and problems related to drug addiction have remained more or less stable since the late 1980s. Addiction to cannabis has been relatively rare in the Netherlands (see Table 10.1). Of the 675,000 regular cannabis users in the Netherlands, approximately 2,500 (0.4 percent of cannabis users) have cannabis addiction problems. Some 25,000 people are addicted to hard drugs. Some 60,000 Dutch use cocaine, 30,000 Dutch use Ecstasy, and another 30,000 use amphetamines. The number of deaths due to accidental and other poisoning by opiates and other narcotics has been stable at about sixty deaths per year. Compared to the number of deaths by alcohol, deaths from heroin and narcotic overdoses are rare. There are approximately 350,000 alcoholics in the Netherlands; of these, 1,600 die from alcoholism or alcohol-related disorders each year.

The Dutch Model of Harm Reduction

Critics of the Dutch approach to dealing with the drug problem point out that there is still a serious drug problem in the Netherlands. Proponents agree that the Dutch drug problem has not disappeared, but in comparison with the other European countries that use a prohibition model, Holland has less of a drug problem.

Even so, the Dutch do not tolerate the negative systems and cultures associated with illegal drug use. To the Dutch, hard-drug use constitutes a major social and administrative problem. Their data show that it is a small number, about 20 percent of hard-core drug addicts, who are responsible for the majority of problems reported to authorities. These problem addicts commit a large number of property offenses in order to obtain the money to buy drugs. Contrary to expectations, however, easy access to methadone as a substitute for heroin has not done much to reduce crime among this group. They have an extremely unconventional lifestyle, in which living on the streets, using multiple drugs, and crime are common. They engage in the sale of drugs, drug-related crime, and antisocial behavior, like throwing away used needles in public places. These behaviors, considered a nuisance, are particularly aggravating to residents in socially disadvantaged neighborhoods in the big cities. In a few cases, residents of drug-infested neighborhoods have taken the law into their own hands by physically driving addicts from their neighborhoods (and closing their streets to drug tourists) (Netherlands Ministry of Health, Welfare and Sports, 1999b).

The Basic Principles of the Opium Act

The Opium Act of 1919, which was amended in 1928 and 1976, regulates the production, distribution, and consumption of psychoactive substances. Possession, commercial distribution, production, import and export, and advertising the sale or distribution of all drugs is punishable by law. Since 1985 this has also covered predatory activities for trafficking hard drugs. Based on the principle that everything should be done to prevent drug users from entering the criminal underworld, the use of drugs is not an offense under Dutch law.

Netherlands' Opium Act draws a distinction between hard drugs (e.g., heroin, cocaine, and Ecstasy), which pose an unacceptable hazard to health, and soft drugs (e.g., hashish and marijuana), which constitute a far less serious hazard. The possession of drugs is an offense in Holland; however, the possession of a small quantity of soft drugs for personal use is a minor one (Spuit and van Laar, 1997).

Importing and exporting drugs are the most serious offenses under the provisions of the Opium Act, although manufacturing, selling, and attempting to import drugs are also offenses. As is the case in other countries, the cultivation of hemp is prohibited, except for certain agricultural purposes (e.g., to form windbreaks and for the production of rope). New legislation is currently being drafted to raise the maximum penalty for commercial hemp production from two to four years in prison (Spuit and van Laar, 1997).

HISTORY OF ALCOHOL AND DRUG ABUSE IN THE NETHERLANDS

In the 1960s and 1970s the use of drugs such as cannabis and opiates increased markedly among the young in Western Europe and North America. Since then, levels of consumption of the various types of drugs in these countries have fluctuated considerably, and there have been fads in consumption from one drug to another. In some countries, total use has increased; in others, including the Netherlands, drug consumption appears to have stabilized at the level it reached around 1980 (Netherlands Ministry of Health, Welfare and Sports 1999a).

Even so, the use of cannabis and opiates has not fallen dramatically, let alone been eradicated in the Netherlands. Those who hoped that a firm government policy would achieve this end have been disappointed. However, given previous international efforts to control or stop trafficking in illegal products or services, government intervention could only be expected to have a limited effect. The Dutch objectives were modest: They wanted to stop a drug problem that continued to increase despite tougher drug laws, and they wanted to reduce the contact between the criminal element and soft-drug users. Drug use was and is considered to be a health and social problem that needs to be controlled, not prohibited (Netherlands Ministry of Health, Welfare and Sports, 1999a).

In pragmatic terms, the Dutch drug policy has achieved some success. The use of drugs of all types is roughly the same now as it was in 1980. From a medical point of view, drug consumption has not become a more serious problem. The use of nicotine and alcohol takes an incomparably higher toll on people's health in the Netherlands (as indeed it does in other parts of the Western world) than the use of all sanctioned drugs covered by the Opium Act. Following the recommendations of the Working Party on Narcotics in 1972, the Dutch government based future drug policies on the idea that using illegal drugs in and of itself was an acceptable risk to society. The unacceptable risk to society depended on how the drugs were used and the extent of their use (Netherlands Ministry of Health, Welfare and Sports, 1997).

The Development of Coffee Shops

The Dutch drug policy has been in place since parliament's 1976 acceptance of the recommendation of the Baan Committee's 1972 report. The committee was headed by Pieter A.H. Baan, a psychiatrist and expert in addiction rehabilitation who was, at the time, serving in the Dutch Office of Mental Health. The Baan Committee's report proposed distinguishing between schedule I drugs (those that present an unacceptable risk—hard drugs such as heroin, cocaine, LSD, and amphetamines) and schedule II drugs (soft drugs or cannabis products, such as hashish and marijuana believed to be less dangerous). Essentially, parliament decriminalized the possession of 30 grams of marijuana (calculated to meet an average smoker's needs for three months). At the same time, the parliamentarians agreed to continue the fight against both domestic and international trafficking in the more dangerous schedule I drugs (Collins, 1999).

Shortly after accepting the commission's primary recommendation, parliament authorized the commercialization of cannabis products through their open sale in a network of licensed coffee shops. The shops were subject to a number of legal constraints, such as not allowing the sale of more than 30 grams to a customer, no sales of hard drugs on the premises, no advertising, no sales to minors, and no operations within 500 meters (650 yards) of a school. Out of respect for Holland's international treaty obligations, the import, export, production, or sale of cannabis products outside the coffee shops remained illegal (Netherlands Ministry of Health, Welfare and Sports, 1999a).

Cultivation of *Nederwiet* in Netherlands

In 1976, when the Dutch allowed cannabis to be sold legally in licensed coffee shops, importing marijuana into Holland was still illegal under the nation's international treaty obligations. Subsequently, the Dutch began to grow marijuana themselves. *Nederwiet*, as homegrown marijuana is known in the Netherlands, is reported to have a smooth taste and to be very potent. Marijuana smoke of any kind, however, is known to be harsh and impossible for noncigarette smokers to hold in their lungs without a good bit of practice and effort. Compared to other marijuana *Nederwiet* may be called smooth, but it is still very harsh. At any rate, many that smoke marijuana maintain that *Nederwiet* is one of the best on the market. In the year 2000, *Nederwiet* is more potent than when the coffee shops opened in 1979. Over the years, by using better cultivation methods and cross-pollination, *Nederwiet* has increased in potency. When the coffee shops opened, the amount of delta-nine-tetrahydro-cannabinol (THC) (the intoxicating chemical in cannabis), was about 5 percent. By 2000, the THC content of *Nederwiet* was allegedly as high as 30 percent. Moreover, it was estimated that 70 percent of the cannabis smoked in Holland's 1,500 coffee shops was *Nederwiet* (Cohen, 1996).

Nederwiet Production

What is as striking as the increase in potency is the rapid increase in the amount of homegrown *Nederwiet*. When the coffee shops came into existence in 1979, *Nederwiet*, for all practical purposes, did not exist. Today, according to Professor Adrian Jansen of the economics faculty of the University of Amsterdam, the annual *Nederwiet* harvest is estimated to be somewhere around 100 tons a year. A portion of the crop of *Nederwiet* is exported to other countries, which is illegal and results in a jail term for traffickers (Dufour, van der Haar, and van der Hoeven, 1996).

Decriminalizing the sale of marijuana in Holland led to the development of a sizable business sector. According to the Dutch Ministry of Justice, the *Nederwiet* industry employs about 20,000 people. The overall commercial value of the industry, including not only the growth and sale of the plant itself, but also the export of high-potency *Nederwiet* seeds to the rest of Europe and the United States, is 20 billion Dutch guilders (about $10 billion U.S.). The illegal export of cannabis today brings in far more money than the more traditional Dutch crop, the tulip (Dufour, van der Haar, and van der Hoeven, 1996).

Under Dutch law, anyone may possess five plants for personal use. Officials, however, estimate that the *Nederwiet* crop (100 tons) is produced by between 25,000 and 30,000 growers. Most of these people grow their cannabis indoors, in a garage, in a basement, or in a back room. On the average, each grower is producing between seven and eight pounds of *Nederwiet* per year. In a year, an individual could easily grow two crops (Spuit and van Laar, 1997).

SUBSTANCE ABUSE IN THE NETHERLANDS TODAY

Political Views and Public Policies

The harm-reduction drug policies, based on a health-focused model and adopted by Dutch legislators, led to a large-scale methadone program and a needle-exchange system. Both programs started in the Netherlands in the 1970s. What is interesting and important when studying policy is the effect of the harm-reduction model on the Dutch people during the AIDS epidemic in the 1980s, ten years after the methadone and needle-exchange programs started. The main aim of the drug policy in the Netherlands was to protect the health of individual users, the people around them, and society as a whole. Protecting the health of the Netherlands' young people was a priority (Cohen, 1996). The Dutch drug policies are based on a health model; the U.S. drug policies are based on a prohibition model.

The methadone programs were designed to enable addicts who participated in the programs to lead a reasonably normal life, without his or her addiction causing a nuisance to his or her family or the community. Needle-exchange programs were started to help prevent the transmission of diseases such as hepatitis B through dirty, infected needles. This service also provides counseling (Netherlands Ministry of Health, Welfare and Sports, 1997).

In the 1980s, when HIV/AIDS was spreading through the needle-using addict communities at an alarming rate, Holland was proportionately affected by HIV/AIDS among their needle-using addict community. HIV/AIDS spread so rapidly among needle-using addicts because of the legal sanctions in most countries preventing the legal purchase of hypodermic needles. However, once the "dirty needle" link was made between drug use and HIV/AIDS, Dutch addicts stopped using dirty needles. Since the 1980s, Dutch addicts have had access to clean needles supplied by the government. Consequently, the Dutch drug policies also appear to have had a positive impact in reducing new cases of HIV/AIDS in the 1980s and 1990s. The Dutch AIDS prevention program was equally successful. In Europe, as a whole in 1997, an average of 39.2 percent of AIDS victims use hypodermic needles. In the Netherlands, the percentage of AIDS victims who used hypodermic needles was as low as 10.5 percent (Netherlands Ministry of Health, Welfare and Sports, 1997).

Our Liberal Drug Policy Has Been a Failure

As might be expected, the people of Holland are not 100 percent behind this drug policy, even if the evidence demonstrates a reduction in the number of teens exposed to hard drugs and the criminal element that sells them, and even if the number of cases of HIV/AIDS infection in the addict community is lower than in the rest of Europe. "Our liberal drug policy has been a failure, but its advocates are so rooted to their convictions they can't bring themselves to admit it," stated Dr. Franz Koopman, director of De Hoop (The Hope) drug rehabilitation center in Dordecht, Netherland.

First, we banalized cannabis use. We have left our kids with the idea that it's perfectly alright to smoke it, and from there it was an easy step for them to move to the notion that it's also okay to use mind-altering substances like ecstasy. It is that mentality that is behind the explosion in the use of these synthetics we have had in the last three years, and [it] is a grave peril to this country just as it is to the rest of Europe. (Collins, 1999, p. 82)

The probation approach for dealing with the problem of substance abuse has its proponents within Holland but, by and large, it is the policy position of the rest of the nations of the world. Oddly enough, however, there is not the same outcry to prohibit the production and consumption of alcohol, coffee, and tea to name a few of the soft drugs available to young people around the world.

Social Views, Customs, and Practices

Being known as the country that legalized drugs is irritating not only to politicians but to the Dutch people in general. They are often the brunt of claims that Holland is the cause of the drug problems experienced by their neighbors. Nothing annoys the Dutch more than drug tourism.

Drug Tourism

Drug tourism is more common along the border with Belgium and Germany, but it is also seen in towns in the interior of the country. Some tourists bring their own drugs to use while in the Netherlands, and others take them home across the border. The problem, as the Dutch see it, is the hard-drug tourist. Too often, hard-drug tourism has gone hand in hand with drug runners and users who have created intolerable annoyances in residential areas, town centers, and public parks (Netherlands Ministry of Health, Welfare and Sports, 1999b).

The battle against drug tourism in the middle to late 1990s resulted in numerous arrests. In 1994 over 800 drug tourists and drug traffickers were arrested. However, a police crackdown in one area simply resulted in the drug traffickers and drug tourists moving to another area of Holland. The repressive policy aimed at discouraging foreign drug tourism continues. At the same time, more effort is being made to investigate and prosecute the leading pushers of hard drugs in Holland (Netherlands Ministry of Health, Welfare and Sports, 1999b).

Cutting the Number of Coffee Shops in 1995

Recognizing that a number of coffee houses had become involved in selling hard drugs as well as soft drugs, in 1995 a joint policy of the Dutch Ministries of Foreign Affairs, Health, Welfare and Sport, Justice, and the Interior cut down on the number of coffee shops. The policy also reduced the amount that could be sold to one individual from 30 grams to 5 grams. In Rotterdam, the number was cut from over a 100 coffee houses to 65. Officials distinguished between "good" and "bad" coffee shops. Often the bad coffee shops were owned by Moroccan or East European owners, who more often did not follow the strict coffee shop laws (Netherlands Ministry of Health, Welfare and Sports, 1999b).

Hard Drugs in Holland

Because of public exposure of the heroin and cocaine addicts in Holland, and the "loser" image of hard-drug addicts in prevention messages, the number of young people using heroin and cocaine continued to decline into the late 1990s. The picture of old addicts, unkempt and pathetic, living in filth and poverty, is believed to be a compelling argument against the use of heroin.

As important to the success of the Dutch drug policy, and the psychological battle to reduce dangerous drug use by young people, is the approach used by authorities to deal with people addicted to hard drugs. Because Dutch authorities do not prosecute drug addicts simply for using drugs, and because the state provides methadone as a substitute for heroin to anyone who asks for it, the drug addict's lifestyle and addiction are not regarded by the young Dutch as a form of social or cultural rebellion. European advocates of liberalizing drug laws, such as Paul Flynn, a Welsh Labour member of the British Parliament, make the point that by making cannabis freely available to their youth, the Dutch have turned many of their young people away from heroin (Collins, 1999). And, based on good data, it is true that, in Holland, the heroin-addicted population is growing older.

Treatment in Prison

Hard-drug addicts in Dutch jails made up about 10 percent of the prisoners in the 1970s, but 50 percent or more in 1995. Among clients in jail who are registered with the Consultation Bureaus for Alcohol and Drugs (CAD), about 50 percent were prosecuted for property offenses. Since there have been more legally available hard drugs and methadone, and the penalties have been reduced for activities related to drug addiction, prosecution of CAD clients for drug dealing have dropped from more than 30 percent in 1989 to 13 percent in 1995. In the last years of the twentieth century, the Amsterdam police reported declining criminal rates, mainly due to a decrease in petty crimes to obtain drug money. Street robbery, house break-ins, auto theft, and picking pockets were all down about 20 percent between 1993 and 1996 (Bovens, 1996).

Rapid Increase in Ecstasy

The drug scene in Holland, like the rest of the developed countries, shifts from one drug to another. At the beginning of the twenty-first century, there was a rapid increase in the production and consumption of Ecstasy and amphetamines. Dutch Prime Minister Willem Kok, in 1996, told his Ministry of Justice to "show our European neighbors we take this ecstasy problem seriously and that we're going to do something about it." The result was the creation in 1997 of an interregional police task force, the

Unit against Synthetic Drugs (USD), which employs sixty police officers to collect a database and work with other police forces (Collins, 1999). At this time, little was known about the long-term consequences of sustained Ecstasy use. One of the more scientific studies on the effect of Ecstasy was published in October 1998 in the British medical journal *The Lancet*. The study was conducted by the Biological Psychiatry Branch of the National Institute of Mental Health in Bethesda, Maryland. Although the sample was small and the results were thus flawed, there were clear indications that prolonged, regular use of Ecstasy could result in irreversible damage to the serotonin receptors in the brain. The consequence could be that some of today's heavy Ecstasy users might find themselves experiencing chronic depression later in life. Or, Ecstasy could act like other serotonin inhibitors, which are used to treat depression. After the person stops using the antidepressant drug, the body reestablishes its serotonin equilibrium (McCann et al., 1998). To accomplish its goal of dealing with the Ecstasy problem, Dutch officials planned to increase prevention programs and arrest and prosecute the traffickers and producers (Netherlands Ministry of Health, Welfare and Sports, 1999a).

The Impact of Legalization on Teenagers

Dutch teenagers can buy beer and wine when they reach the age of sixteen; however, they cannot legally buy marijuana at coffee shops until they are eighteen years of age (Spuit and van Laar, 1997). According to Holland's official statistics, the Dutch murder rate is 80 percent below the U.S. rate. They have a lower rate of hard-drug addiction and even a lower rate of marijuana use than the United States. For the most part, Holland was spared the crack cocaine epidemic that followed the suppression of marijuana in the United States in the 1980s. Over the years, data that have been collected indicate cannabis use patterns among Dutch teenagers typically begin at about twelve or thirteen years of age, increase until the age of sixteen or seventeen, and then decline. For the Dutch, this indicates that teens experiment with cannabis and then quit using it (Spuit and van Laar, 1997). The Dutch believe that this positive outcome is directly related to the health model used in Holland.

Addiction Treatment in the Netherlands

The Dutch treatment system began in the early 1900s, by and large as a reaction to widespread alcoholism in the Netherlands. Treatment was a part of the initiatives of alcohol activists and prohibitionists. Psychiatric hospitals set up specialized residential treatment clinics for alcoholics. The outpatient treatment system (ambulatory system of the CADs), consisting of social-medical centers for treating the alcohol-dependent person, was founded in the 1920s. The CADs were subsidized by the Ministry of Justice, so they also functioned as probation institutes (Spuit and van Laar, 1997).

The Sum and Substance of the Treatment Model

The sum and substance of this health policy was best stated by the former head of the Department of Social Psychiatry of the Amsterdam Municipal Health Service, Dr. Wignand Mulder (1981): "If cure is not possible, not doing harm is the next target" (Denks, Hoekstra and Kaplan, 1998, p.2).

Dutch politicians continue to support the policy direction. The last major government memorandum, *Drug Policy in the Netherlands: Continuity and Change* (1999) states,

Given the relatively good results which have been achieved, we do not believe that there is any reason for a fundamental re-examination of drugs policy in the Netherlands, which is primarily geared to control the harm done to people's health. (Netherlands Ministry of Health, Welfare and Sports, 1999b)

The goal of providing a livable and safe environment for its entire people is among the highest priorities in the Netherlands. To accomplish this, the Netherlands has invested an extra 60 million guilders ($35 million U.S.) in programs designed to reduce drug-related nuisance crimes and in developing facilities for the treatment and rehabilitation of the addicts who cause the nuisance. Addicted offenders are now given the option of detoxification treatment or serving a prison sentence (Netherlands Ministry of Health, Welfare and Sports, 1999b).

Prevention and the Care and Treatment of the Addict

The prevention of drug use and addiction are integral to Dutch drug policies. The treatment of addicts is also a focal point of the Dutch policies. The goal is to have treatment available to anyone who asks for it.

1. Prevention. Prevention programming is an important component of the Dutch drug policy. Drug-prevention programs at the school level are a major focus of the effort to discourage drug use. Additionally, mass media campaigns are developed to reach a larger public audience. Because of constantly changing drug preferences, trends, and fads, monitoring changes in drug use plays an important role in Holland's prevention efforts. Because of these studies, more prevention messages and programming are geared to reach the vulnerable groups who run the risk of serious addiction problems. In the late 1990s, those groups were identified as foreign youth and multiple drug users (Bovens, 1996).

2. Care. The protection of the health of drug users is another major focus of the Dutch drug policy. To meet this goal, a wide range of facilities are available. The Netherlands spends more than 300 million guilders (approximately $175 million U.S.) a year on facilities for addicts. Over half of this amount is spent on the hard-drug problem. There are twelve clinics for the treatment of addicts, and the capacity has been increased from 500 treatment slots in 1980 to approximately 2,000 treatment slots in 1995. During the 1990s, accessibility of drug treatment increased and reached an estimated 75 percent of all addicts. Their aim is to reach as many addicts as possible and to support them in their efforts to rehabilitate themselves, or to limit the risks caused by their drug habit. Social rehabilitation is an essential element of the Dutch drug policy (Netherlands Ministry of Health, Welfare and Sports, 1997).

Dutch Drug Treatment

The Netherlands has an extensive network of specialized institutions to treat alcoholics and addicts for their dependency. Treatment varies according to client needs. Treatment might consist of outpatient, inpatient, or a mix of both. They treat alcohol, drug, and gambling dependencies. Treatment of addiction is clearly different from treatment provided as a general mental health service.

The Dutch approach to drug treatment is similar to the approach used in the United States. The most intense treatment would include inpatient treatment under the care of a psychiatrist. However, most treatment programs would include residential treatment followed by outpatient treatment that might include methadone maintenance. The approach to treatment also includes "street-corner" work, relief work, crisis intervention, counseling, prevention work, day and open-door centers, and study, work, and housing projects. A number of projects are aimed at specific groups such as Moroccans and Surinamese and at certain categories of clients such as heroin addicts, drug-using prostitutes, and children of addicted mothers. Prevention and treatment is provided to individuals and groups according to local environmental circumstances and priorities (Kooyman, 1992).

For severely addicted clients, treatment may consist of detoxification and a brief stay of several weeks; it could consist of a short stay of up to three months; or it could mean an even longer stay. Treatment at any level is followed by aftercare at an outpatient clinic. Eleven independent services and nine departments of general psychiatric hospitals specialize in dependency care. The total of 900 treatment beds for the entire country of the Netherlands is smaller than the addiction bed capacity of South Florida. Much of the long-term drug treatment of addicts in Holland takes place in drug-free therapeutic communities similar to those used in the United States. This treatment model, which typically requires abstinence, uses phases that vary from an intensive program to less restrictive care. Clinical program evaluations that focus on outcomes, retention of patients, and comorbidity in drug addicts in treatment have helped to improve the treatment outcomes in Dutch drug-treatment centers (Kooyman, 1992).

Self-Help Groups

A number of self-help organizations also play a role. Alcoholics Anonymous (AA) has been active in the Netherlands for more than fifty years. Recovering drug addicts participate in Narcotics Anonymous (NA) groups which follow the traditions of AA. The National Foundation for Parents of Drug Addicts and the National Point of Support for Drug Users also operate throughout the Netherlands, with self-help and policy advocacy as their objectives. As well, associations of former clients of therapeutic communities provide aftercare services as well as support for the community programs. The relationship between self-help groups and the professional institutions is good. The professional institutions often provide meeting rooms and secretarial assistance to the self-help groups. The advocacy groups also play an important role in stimulating the professional institutions to try out prevention and treatment innovations (Derks, Hoekstra, and Kaplan, 1998).

In 1993 the government set up intervention programs to diminish drug-related nuisance and crime: The addicted offender has a choice between strict punishment or treatment. Additionally, in many prisons, cellblocks are being established as drug-free areas for inmates who are in recovery, and more places in residential treatment facilities are being provided for criminal clients in residential treatment programs (Derks, Hoekstra, and Kaplan, 1998).

THE FUTURE OF SUBSTANCE ABUSE IN THE NETHERLANDS

Dutch officials are proposing a plan to change many of the remaining drug laws which are responsible for filling Dutch jails and prisons. Official estimates suggest that as many as 50 percent of jail beds would be freed up if people were not incarcerated for activities undertaken to maintain their drug habits. When Dutch authorities arrest foreign drug addicts, the courts are now allowing them to return to their homelands for drug treatment.

Because the Dutch believe that their drug policies have been so successful, initiatives to decriminalize hard-drug use and addiction can be expected. Future policies will decriminalize the distribution of hard drugs to addicted Dutch citizens. In the near future in Holland,

1. Hard drugs will be sold legally to Dutch citizens who are eighteen years of age or older (the same age required for alcohol and marijuana).

2. Potential hard-drug buyers will have to submit to identification and registration to buy hard drugs legally.

3. A National Drug Agency will be developed to provide the buyer with a "drug pass." This pass could contain a code with personal data. Any purchase of drugs

could be registered with a central database. The drug pass could be similar to an ATM card and would not be transferable.

4. The drug pass would allow the user a predetermined amount of a certain drug for a certain time period, or would allow a combination of several drugs for multidrug users.

5. If the user should want more drugs than the regular drug pass allows, he would be able to buy them with a special permit. In such cases, the only restrictions placed on the sale of additional drugs to an addict would be those restrictions that would prevent resale.

6. The Dutch Drug Agency will determine the points of sale (i.e., drug shops) just as it controls the point of sale of cannabis in coffee shops. If resale becomes a problem, drug-user rooms will be set up where addicts will use their drugs in the shop where they buy their drugs.

7. The Dutch Drug Agency will set the price of the hard drugs sold in the drug shops to compete with illegal drug sales.

8. The drug pass (for Dutch citizens only) would also discourage an invasion from foreign hard-drug users, as well as quell some of the objections from the EU against the Dutch policy.

9. After studying the experience with a method of supplying hard drugs to addicts, do not be surprised if Holland makes its findings available to other nations in the hopes that surrounding countries will decide to decriminalize the production and sale of hard drugs so that hard distribution can be gradually normalized and be brought in line with the system that is used to sell soft drugs in Holland (Derks, Hoekstra, Kaplan, 1998, p. 37).

Proposed Solutions and Strategies

In addition to changing many of the drug laws, the Dutch are requesting their neighbors to look at the positive effect that decriminalizing soft drugs can have on their young people, not to mention the cost of arrest, prosecution, and incarceration. In another, unique approach, the Dutch are also planning to force coffee shop sellers to reduce the THC level of marijuana so that it is not stronger than the illegal marijuana that tourists can buy in their own countries. The same strategy was used with producers of whiskies and other liquors in the United States; these alcoholic beverages are limited to 80 proof alcohol without a special permit.

Results of the Dutch Drug Policy

Based on the numbers of those who have been harmed by the worldwide substance-abuse problem, the Dutch believe their policy approach has been a success. In 1995, 2.4 drug-related deaths per million were reported among the Dutch. In the same year, France reported 9.5 deaths per million; Germany, 20; Sweden, 23.5; and Spain, 27.1. Based on the 1995 report of the

European Monitoring Center for Drugs and Drug Addiction in Lisbon, Holland had the lowest number of drug-related deaths per million in Europe (Netherlands Ministry of Health, Welfare and Sports, 1997).

The Dutch drug policies also appear to have had a positive impact in reducing new cases of HIV/AIDS. The Dutch AIDS-prevention program was equally successful. In Europe as a whole, an average of 39.2 percent of AIDS victims are intravenous drug users. In the Netherlands, the percentage of AIDS victims who are intravenous drug users is as low as 10.5 percent (Netherlands Ministry of Health, Welfare and Sports, 1997).

The number of addicts in the Netherlands has been stable at 25,000 since 1980. This number of Dutch addicts is approximately the same as the numbers found in Germany, Sweden, and Belgium. In Holland, the average age of the hard-drug addict is thirty-six years. The data also indicate that there were fewer young narcotic addicts in the Netherlands, in the year 2000, than in 1980 (Netherlands Ministry of Health, Welfare and Sports, 1997).

CONCLUSIONS

Although critics point out that there is still a serious drug problem in the Netherlands, advocates for the Dutch model point out that there is also a serious problem with alcohol, which is also sold legally in the Netherlands. Advocates say that the goal of the Dutch drug policy is not to wipe out drug use, but to slow or stop the movement from soft drugs to hard drugs. In the 1970s their scientists did not believe that drug use could be eliminated without doing great damage to the soul of Dutch society. Their goals were more modest. The goal of the policy was to separate the soft-drug market from the hard-drug market and all of the problems that go with a hard-drug market. They also wanted to reduce the harm to their youth who experimented with drugs, particularly soft drugs. The question of harm and drug use as a threat to society was reconsidered. Smoking marijuana did not seem as harmful to the individual as the harm done to the individual by spending twenty years in jail for smoking marijuana.

The scientist and treatment professionals who helped shape the Dutch model and the Dutch drug policies in the mid-1970s made what has turned out to be a good decision for the Dutch people in respect to using a health model to control the spread of addiction and to deal with the upsurges in drug use which have occurred over the last twenty-five years. It has also been a policy that has helped maintain one of the smallest percentages of HIV/AIDS cases among intravenous drug users in the world.

As it turns out, the Dutch have achieved many of the goals that they hoped to accomplish twenty-five years ago with their drug policy legislation. There is a separation of the soft- and hard-drug markets. Cannabis has been easy to buy in coffee shops for twenty-five years without any unacceptable increase in problems or in the use of cannabis in Holland or in neighboring countries. Extremely important is the drug policy's influence on hard-drug addicts. The number of hard-drug addicts stabilized in 1980 and continued over the next twenty years at about the same level. Moreover, the Netherlands has had fewer drug-related deaths than in most other EU countries. In the mid 1990s, other EU countries began to employ decriminalization laws on soft drugs as an alternative to building additional prisons for their young people. Many have come to view adolescent fascination with drugs as being related to the adolescent's need to differentiate himself or herself from his or her parents and others who profoundly influence their lives. The goal of parents, the goal of a caring community, and the goal of a caring state is to help the adolescent move through this period of searching for an identity and teenage rebellion. Arresting, prosecuting, and incarcerating teenagers and young adults who get caught up in playing out the rebellious theme of *Easy Rider* or a television docudrama is not dealing with the drug problem. Its only effect is to inflict grave harm on the teens and young adults who are unlucky enough to be caught by the authorities.

REFERENCES

Bovens, R. (Ed.). (1996). *Justice and care*. Utrecht: Dutch Association of Addiction Treatment Centers.

Cohen, P. (1996, March). *The case of the two Dutch drug policy commissions: An exercise in harm reduction*. Toronto, Canada: Addiction Research Foundation. Paper presented at the 5th International Conference on the Reduction of Drug Related Harm.

Collins, L. (1999, May/June). Holland's half-baked drug experiment. *Essays*, Washington, D.C.: Council on Foreign Relations, Inc., p. 82. Copyright© 1999 by Council on Foreign Relations Inc.

Derks, J.T.M., Hoekstra, M.J., and Kaplan, C.D. (1998). Integrating care, cure, and control: The drug treatment system in the Netherlands. In Klingemann, H., and Hunt, G. (Eds.). *Drug treatment systems in an international perspective: Drugs, demons, and delinquents* (pp. 201–209). Thousand Oaks, CA: Sage Publications.

Dufour, R., van der Haar, J., and van der Hoeven, R. (1996). *Drug control through legalisation: A plan for regulation of the drug problem in the Netherlands*. Hamingen, the Netherlands: Dutch Drug Policy Foundation.

Encarta Desk Encyclopedia (1998). Netherlands. Microsoft Corporation on CD-ROM.

Kooyman, M. (1992). *The therapeutic community for addicts: Intimacy, parent involvement and treatment success*. Amsterdam: Swets & Zeitlinger.

McCann, U.D., Szabo, Z., Scheffel, U., Dannals, R.F., and Ricaurte, G.A. (1998). Positron emission tomographic evidence of toxic effect of MDMA ("Ecstasy") on brain serotonin neurons in human beings. *Lancet, 352* 4 (9138) 1433–1437.

Netherlands Board of Tourism. (2000). *General information*. Leidschendam: Au-

thor. Retrieved on November 11, 2000, from the World Wide Web: http://
www.visitholland.com/

Netherlands Ministry of Health, Welfare and Sports. (1997). *Drug policy in the
Netherlands: Progress report September 1997*. The Hague: Author. Retrieved
on November 16, 2000, from the World Wide Web: http://www.netherlands-
embassy.org/c_hltdru.html

————. (1999a). *Drug policy in the Netherlands: Progress report September 1997—
September 1999*. The Hague: Author. Retrieved on November 16, 2000, from
the World Wide Web: http://www.netherlands-embassy.org/c_hltdru.html

————. (1999b). *Drug policy in the Netherlands: Continuity and change*. The Hague:
Author. Retrieved on November 1, 2000, from the World Wide Web: http://
www.minvws.nl/

Newton, G. (1978). *The Netherlands*. New York: Westview Press.

Spuit, I.P., & van Laar, M.W. (1997). *Fact sheet 7: Cannabis policy, update*. Utrecht:
Trimbos Institute.

11

RUSSIA

Kathryn C. Shafer

INTRODUCTION

The recent political changes in the Commonwealth of Independent States (CIS), formerly called the Union of Soviet Socialist Republics (USSR), and the collapse of the Soviet system have radically altered and worsened the lives of its people. This change for the worse is due to severe economic hardship, loss of moral values, lack of faith in the government, lack of efficient medical care, increasing infant mortality, and consumption of cheap, nondistilled, and often toxic poison beverages (Segal, 2000).

These changes have led to international concern and media exposure. This chapter examines the role and impact of alcohol and substance use in a collapsed political nation. These rapid and extreme economic, political, and social shifts have given rise to deep apathy and lack of hope for the future. Pessimism and social depression breed the environment and culture for illicit drug use.

A Brief Profile of Russia

Even after the break-up of the Soviet Union, the Russian Federation (Rossiskaya Federatsiy), in geographical size, is still the largest country in the world. Russia covers more than 11 percent of the earth's surface (17,075,200 square kilometers, or 6,592,770 square miles). Of that, only 7.8 percent is arable land. Russia extends north to the Arctic Ocean and east to the Pacific Ocean. This location gives Russia the longest continuous coastline (37,650 kilometers, or 23,400 miles) of any country in the world. Even so, Russia has almost no year-round oceanic ports because most of the coastal waters are frozen for most of the year.

Permafrost, or permanently frozen subsoil, which is found throughout the northern region, provides limited sustenance to plants. Forests, which cover 45 percent of Russia, account for nearly 25 percent of the world's forest area.

Russia contains the greatest mineral reserves of any country in the world. It is especially rich in mineral fuels, including petroleum and natural gas.

The People of Russia

The majority of the 146,861,022 people (1998 estimate) live in European Russia. Although more than 100 nationalities make up the population, Russians account for 82 percent. The official language is Russian. Minorities include Tatars, Ukrainians, Chuvash, Belarussian, Bashkir, and Chechen.

Russian Orthodox Christianity is the primary religion, with an estimated 35 million adherents. The Russian Orthodox Church has played a major role in Russian history that goes back more than 1,100 years.

The Russian population has been shrinking since 1992; it could fall to about 120 million by 2050. It fell by nearly 500,000 in 1996 (McRae, 1997). Population figures in mid-1995, released by the Ministry of Labor, indicate that between 1960 and 1995 about 66 percent of Russia's small villages (those with fewer than 1,000 residents) disappeared. Of the 24,000 that remained in the mid-1990s, more than 50 percent of the population was older than sixty-five years of age (Traynor, 2000).

Education

The Russia Federation inherited a well-developed system of education from the Soviet Union. The Soviet government operated virtually all the schools in Russia. It had an extensive network of preschool, elementary, secondary, and post-secondary schools. The Soviet educational philosophy was simple. The teacher's job was to transmit standardized materials organized around socialist ethics. The student's job was to memorize those materials.

Soviet Communist ethics stressed the primacy of the collective over the interests of the individual. Consequently, creativity and individualism were not valued in the Soviet system of education. Even before the fall of Communist Russia, the educational reform programs in the 1980s called for new curricula, textbooks, and teaching methods. The idea was to develop schools that could better equip Soviet students to deal with the modern, technologically driven economy that Soviet leaders believed would be the trend in the future. However, because of a lack of funding, educational facilities generally were inadequate, overcrowding was common, and equipment and materials were in short supply. The schools and universities could not supply the skilled labor needed in almost every sector of the economy.

At the same time, Russian young people became increasingly cynical about the Marxist-Leninist philosophy, as well as the stifling of self-expression and individual responsibility.

The collapse of the Soviet system and glasnost did what the educational reforms in the 1980s could not do. The collapse opened the door for change in the curriculum. These changes included the teaching of previously banned literary works and a reinterpretation of Soviet and Russian history. In 1995, 2.21 percent of government expenditures went to education.

Economy

Russia's economy was severely crippled when it moved from the Communist system, where prices are controlled by the central government, to a market economy, where prices are determined by industry and by the supply and demand of products. Although the move toward a market economy was met with widespread resistance, it did not stop the economic change from taking place.

As the market system developed, many people found themselves out of work. Unemployment in 1996 was reported to be 9.3 percent. Another 46.5 million people (31 percent) had incomes below the poverty level. The GDP per person in 1996 was $2,980 (U.S. dollars) (Bureau of European Affairs, 2000).

During this period, many Russians experienced unemployment for the first time. Middle-aged workers particularly found it difficult to adjust to the loss of the cradle-to-grave social security provided by the Soviet system. The gap between Russia's "haves" and "have-nots" continues to grow. In the new economic system, the "haves" are distinguished by skills, audacity, and connections to influential people (Bureau of European Affairs, 2000).

Worker Benefits

Russian law provides numerous protections that meet the needs of adolescent mothers and all women of childbearing age. This legislation merges family policy and employment policy to assist mothers and families. Women who are employed are entitled to paid maternity-leave from seventy days prior to giving birth until seventy days afterward. Despite what may look like generosity from the state, maternity-leave salary and benefits are based on the Russian minimum wage, not on a woman's current wage. This increases the cost of childbearing to the mother and family.

A portion of Russian workers have entitlements to housing, child care, and paid vacations, regardless of their rank within a company. Housing entitlements involve either outright provision of a low-rent apartment, cash, or in-kind housing. Furthermore, occupants obtain an ownership right to the apartment extending beyond their employment and into retirement. They may also have the legal title to the apartment transferred to their own name without paying any purchase price.

The Social Insurance Fund, which administers the payment of benefits, is managed by the largest union organization in Russia, the Federation of Independent Trade Unions of Russia (Federatsiya nezavisimykh profsoyuzov Rossii, or FNPR). Employers contribute 5.4 percent of the total payroll to fund the benefits.

At the end of 1995, some 8,200,000 people were registered as unemployed. The true number is thought to be much higher. In 1998 about 5,000,000 people were unemployed. The "new poor," according to the World Bank, far exceeds the resources available in Russia for social welfare. The Communist system, with all of its problems, provided universal employment. Without a job, able-bodied citizens do not have access to social security benefits. In post-Communist Russia, unemployment and the lack of funding for basic social services are openly acknowledged (Bureau of European Affairs, 2000).

Alcohol, Narcotics, and Tobacco

Russia's rate of alcohol consumption has been among the highest in the world since people started counting. Even so, alcohol consumption continued to increase throughout the 1990s. Alcoholism, particularly among men, is the third leading cause of death after cardiovascular diseases and cancer. Periodic government campaigns to reduce alcoholism have resulted in thousands of deaths from the consumption of illegal alcohol called *samogon* (a homemade vodka similar to American moonshine).

The last campaign to reduce alcoholism was undertaken by Mikhail Gorbachev's administration between 1985 and 1988. The government efforts failed, and public anger over the restrictions on the amount of vodka one could purchase and the increase in the cost of vodka contributed to Gorbachev's failure to win reelection. By 1987 the production of *samogon* had become a large-scale industry, depriving the state of significant tax revenue. When restrictions were eased in 1988, alcohol consumption exceeded the pre-1985 level. One study suggested that between 1987 and 1992 the annual per capita consumption of alcohol rose from about 11 liters (3 gallons) of pure alcohol to 14 liters (3.7 gal.) in 1992. Consumption in the late 1990s was estimated to be 15 liters (4 gal.) of pure alcohol per Russian. The World Health Organization standards suggest that over 8 liters (2 gal.) of pure alcohol per person per year is likely to cause major medical problems. In 1994 about 53,000 Russians died of alcohol poisoning, an increase of about 36,000 over the number of deaths in 1991 (Bureau of European Affairs, 2000).

Crime

In 1994 Russia as a nation averaged eighty-four murders a day. Many of those murders were contract killings attributed to criminal organizations. In 1995 the national crime total exceeded 1.3 million crimes, including 30,600 murders. Crime experts predicted that the murder total would exceed 50,000 per year by the year 2005.

Crime statistics from Moscow in 1995 listed a total of 93,560 crimes. There were 18,500 white-collar crimes—an increase of 8.3 percent over 1994. Swindling increased 67.2 percent, and extortion increased 37.5 percent. Murder and attempted murder increased 1.5 percent; rape, 6.5 percent; burglary, 6.6 percent, burglary accompanied by violence, 20.8 percent, and serious crime by teenagers, 2.2 percent.

After the collapse of the USSR, Russia became a major conduit for the movement of drugs, contraband, and laundered money between Europe and Asia. In 1995 an estimated 150 criminal organizations with transnational links were operating in Russia (Bureau of European Affairs, 2000).

Prisons

Labor camps are strict-regime camps in which inmates work at the most difficult jobs, usually outdoors, and receive meager rations. The system of corrective labor was viewed by Soviet authorities as successful because of the low rate of recidivism.

Prison reforms in 1989 emphasized rehabilitation and attempted to "humanize" the gulag system; nevertheless, few changes were made in the treatment of most prisoners.

In 1994 the estimated prison population was more than 1,000,000 people. Of these about 600,000 were held in labor camps. Of those in labor camps, about 21,600 were women and about 19,000 were adolescents. About 50 percent were imprisoned for violent crimes, 60 percent were repeat offenders, and better than 15 percent were alcoholics or drug addicts. The population of Russian prisons exceeds the capacity of those facilities by an average of 50 percent (Bureau of European Affairs, 2000).

While the average Russian gained greater individual freedom from arbitrary government intrusion after the fall of the USSR, they have been plagued by a crime wave that gets worse with each passing year. Without effective law enforcement, Russian society continues to be an inviting target to criminals in Russia as well as around the world.

VIGNETTE

The court, following a robbery attempt, referred Demitri, a sixteen-year-old boy for counseling. His family consisted of his mother, Mrs. Polsky; Demitri's eighteen-year-old brother; and his stepfather, Mr. Polsky. The family lives in an apartment in a large city. Mr. Polsky works as an engineer at the electric utility; Mrs. Polsky works grooming dogs. Due to hyperactivity and learning problems, Demitri attended a special education class in a public school. He had behavioral outbursts and had difficulty communicating with his stepfather. During the course of therapy with Demitri and his mother, it became apparent that Mr. Polsky had been constantly abusing his wife and children, especially when drinking. The verbal and physical abuses were seen as normal within the family. Although severely beaten at times, Mrs. Polsky denied any family problems and claimed that her husband was just a little too rough.

It was only following an episode in which Mr. Polsky, who was severely drunk, threatened his wife with a knife, and her older son called the police, that Mrs. Polsky admitted that there were problems in her family. She agreed that her husband was probably an alcoholic, but she felt that nothing could be done about it. Mrs. Polsky became teary when talking and asked for help. At this time, she became fearful that her husband would find out that she broke down and told the authorities about the family.

For a short while following this incident, Demitri took a BB gun and began to shoot people on the street from his apartment window. At this point, the mother finally agreed to participate in a women's group, and the stepfather agreed to "do something about his drinking," although he still denied that his alcoholism caused his family any trouble. While "willing" to address the drinking issue, the stepfather is trying to stay sober although he refuses to attend an AA group. He views his hard drinking as appropriate behavior for any Russian man. However, after the counseling, the stepfather was able to stop abusing his stepson and wife.

Demitri was placed in a special school for emotionally disturbed children, and medication was prescribed for him. Very slowly, this family began its recovery process. The healing process is taking much longer than it might have taken owing to the cultural acceptance of hard drinking and domestic violence among Russian families.

OVERVIEW OF SOCIAL ISSUE AND BASIC DEMOGRAPHICS

In a country where a person frequently hears the word *krizis* (crisis) in daily conversation, the following facts will help to describe this environment. Russian life expectancy in the CIS has fallen dramatically in the last ten years (Wines, 2000). The average life span for both sexes (65.9 for both sexes; 59.9 for males, 72.4 for females) is about ten years less than in the United States (77.0 for both sexes; 74.1 for males, 79.7 for females) and is comparable with the levels of life expectancy in Guatemala. Historically, the high incidence of alcoholism in the CIS, that is, the consumption of vodka, remains one of the highest in the world (Segal, 1990), and it is cited as part of the reason for the ongoing health crisis.

Other health-care concerns include massive increases in smoking, increases from suicides from alcohol-related causes, and an almost 60 percent increase in infectious and parasitic diseases (Wines, 2000). Heroin use has proven the deadliest catalyst in this epidemic. The sharp rise in drug use and encouraged needle sharing has spread HIV and AIDS throughout the nation. Today, a region that a decade ago had hardly heard of AIDS and HIV, has recorded 5,000 new cases and more than 8,500 registered drug addicts. These are the official statistics; the true figures could be ten times as great (Wines, 2000). Combine these problems with obsolete medical and social services, and you can begin to grasp the complexity of the situation.

HISTORY OF ALCOHOL AND DRUG USE IN RUSSIA

An exploration of the historical and cultural heritage of excessive drinking and drug use in the CIS reveals that cultural, social, economic, and ideological aspects of the former Soviet Union have implications for therapeutic interventions. Traditionally, the ability to drink large quantities of alcohol was regarded as a sign of manhood and power (Segal, 1987). According to the Kievian Grand Prince Vladimir, "Drinking is the joy of Russia, we cannot do without it" (Segal, 1987, p. 9). Bruised and battered after many years of totalitarian regimes under Lenin, Stalin, Khrushchev, Brezhnev, and other leaders, the Russians have kept their souls buoyant with the ever-present bottle of vodka as a symbol of friendship, community, and hospitality (Kagan and Shafer, 2001).

Discussing alcohol and drug abuse openly as a social problem was forbidden in the years of Stalinism. It was simply regarded as a problem that should simply not occur in a Communist society, and if it was present it was caused by the class enemy or sickness. For this reason, there was no empirical research into drug abuse, and what was known was kept secret from the public. Currently, obtaining recent data on the per capita consumption of alcohol and drug use among the former republics is in its infancy. Information is limited. From the 1950s to the 1970s, a group of Soviet researchers studied the problem of alcoholism through a national survey. However, most of the research was banned, considered propaganda, or censored (Segal, 1990).

Recent Soviet history can be divided into three major periods:

1. The stagnation period or period of slow erosion, associated primarily with the Brezhnev era

2. The period of perestroika and glasnost, or reconstruction and openness (often referred to as the period of dismantling and dismay), under Gorbachev

3. The collapse of communism and the Soviet Union (which was viewed as total disillusionment and consequential disorientation) under the leadership of Boris Yeltsin (Kissin, 1991).

Each of these periods may be examined in terms of their impact on social attitudes, norms, behaviors, and values of the former Soviet citizens.

The period of slow erosion lasted from 1960 until the mid-1980s. This period created a response of significant cognitive conflicts and social isolation. There was mistrust toward authority figures and society while the Soviet individual struggled to maintain Russian family values, traditions, belief, and hope for a better Communist way of life. On the emotional level, hostility was suppressed because it was unsafe to express it openly. Behaviorally, there was a tendency toward general passivity along with attempts to utilize and manipulate the system to obtain basic human needs and services such as food, housing, and medical care. The period of slow erosion, supported by intense rituals of heavy drinking, created an image of the national Russian character. This normalized heavy drinking in the Soviet culture.

Then in the name of reforms that would modernize, humanize, and ultimately save Soviet socialism, Mikhail Gorbachev opened the Iron Curtain and came to power in 1985. Gorbachev provoked the Soviet people to begin taking their destinies into their own hands. He called this vast undertaking "perestroika" and chose this slogan to launch his political campaign to modernize and readapt Soviet socialism without dismantling the system founded by Lenin. The term "perestroika" means "reconstruction," and Gorbachev set out to purify and renew a corrupt and failing socialist system (Traynor, 2000).

The period under perestroika and glasnost, beginning with Gorbachev's rise to power in the mid-1980s, opened previously censored doors to the West. This opening led to the exposure and international awareness of the crimes and abuses of previous political leaders, and the ineffectiveness and poverty supported by the current one. Psychological reactions during this period included disillusionment with the Communist ideology and hope for the emergence of some democratic values. Emotionally, there was much fear and anxiety about the future of Russia as well as feelings of being fooled, manipulated, and victimized by the leaders of their beloved country. Many began to question traditional family values and ties. Many began publicly to express hostility toward authority. Behaviorally, physical confrontation and violence became more prevalent (Kagan & Shafer, 2001). Other social values were challenged during this period, leading to an increase in extramarital affairs, substance abuse, and drug addiction among teenagers. Most recently, open sexual promiscuity, prostitution, and freedom of sexual expression have increased the prevalence of and contributed to the spread of HIV and AIDS (Specter, 1997).

The last seven years in the CIS have been characterized by the collapse of the Soviet system. The cognitive response to this can be described as one of confusion and disorientation. Nationally there is more mistrust of the government and political leadership. Rumors of Boris Yeltsin's ill health, owing to his alcoholism, and widespread corruption, notably the Russian mafia, contributed to the current international political and economic scrutiny. Despite promises to fight corruption, President Vladimir Putin has refused to hand over documents that detail possible money laundering in the billions by Kremlin authorities. Putin's seeming protection and granting Yeltsin immunity from prosecution appear to support the old order (Traynor, 2000).

On an emotional level, the reaction has been one of panic and fear. Behaviorally, there is a hoarding of material possessions and an unprecedented desire and opportunity to flee Russia (Kissin, 1991). The decline of traditional beliefs and values, spiritual emptiness, and interrupted societal development are forcing former Soviets to abandon their roots, ideologies, and ethics in search of new promises and guarantees of quality living. These factors are commonly associated with the escapist reactions that provoke increased alcohol and drug abuse.

SUBSTANCE ABUSE IN RUSSIA TODAY

For many years, bingeing was characterized as the Russian style of drinking. Consumption of large quantities of liquor in short periods, without food and often in solitude, increased the propensity for alcoholism (Kagan, 1992a). An estimated 60 percent of the workforce is said to abuse alcohol, and alcoholism is officially considered the number one health problem among the population (Anderson, 1992). For instance, in 1990, in Saint Petersburg alone there were approximately 80,000 substance abusers, predominantly alcoholics, and 60,000 suicides, many of which were alcohol related. Moreover, there were 19,000 deaths from acute alcohol poisoning; and, of 22,000 murders, 80 percent were alcohol related (Yandow, 1992). In Moscow, about 145,000 patients were registered in the city's narcological (alcohol and drug abuse) treatment centers in 1992. Of these patients, 95 percent were in the most acute stage of the disease, and about 10 percent of all registered patients were women. One in every ten people who requested anonymous treatment was a teenager (interview with Dr. E. Drozdov, the head physician at Moscow's Narcological Hospital No. 17, 1992). Many heavy drinkers, who would be classified as alcohol dependent in Western countries, go undiagnosed and untreated in Russia. The Russians classify a heavy drinker as anyone who goes on drinking binges and is alcohol dependent but does not meet the criteria for a chronic alcoholic. A conservative estimate of chronic alcoholics in Russia is about 15 million; the number of heavy drinkers is three or four times higher (Davis, 1994).

Official Soviet statistics regarding social problems were often unreliable

and, thus, difficult to believe. B.M. Segal (1990) indicates that official figures on alcohol consumption are still only estimates due to reliance on old
Soviet government data. According to the substance-abuse literature, the
most recent accurate account of the state of alcohol and drug treatment is
not based on empirical research but on impressions of professionals traveling
to treatment facilities (Yandow, 1992). However, the estimated per capita
consumption of alcoholic beverages in the USSR in 1985 was eight times
higher than the per capita consumption before the 1917 Russian Revolution, and three times higher than reports on consumption in the United
States. The rate of violent alcohol-related crimes is 10.5 times higher than
that in the United States. The Soviet legal system cannot restrict the illegal
production of *samogon*, or moonshine; the struggle is similar to that during
prohibition in the United States. The reduction of work productivity in the
Russian economy owing to drinking alcohol is estimated to be six times that
in the United States (Segal, 1990).

Currently, there is an escalated use of marijuana, cocaine, heroin, and
prescription drugs. In addition, there are significant increases in sniffing inhalants such as glue, paint, and homemade synthetic drugs by adolescents.

Social Views, Customs, and Practices

In order to understand why Russians drink, it is important to understand
how they drink (Segal, 1990). The Russian drinking style is an expression
of the Russian spirit, courage, escapism, generosity, and even irresponsibility.
The role that alcohol and drug use plays in the life of Russians is unprecedented and cannot be compared to any other culture.

Many times, it has been said that vodka is the lifeblood of the Russian
culture and, conversely, that drinking is the Russian curse. Russia has been
called the land of the endless toast and a nation of male bonding through
the vodka bottle. The Russians are known to have a rigorous social etiquette
requiring that once a bottle of vodka is open, it must be drunk until empty.

The whole notion of autonomy, empowerment, and self-awareness, which
are key ingredients of psychological interventions, were not considered attributes of a healthy mind under the Soviet system. Solidarity with collective
goals and adherence to communal social values were the criteria established
for the development of a healthy personality (Marlin, 1990). Therefore,
individuals received conflicting messages from society. The Soviet system
advocated child-rearing practices that frustrated young citizens' attempts to
attain autonomy and self-reliance.

The insidious process of manipulation within the Soviet totalitarian regime emphasized the loss of individuality and immersion in the societal
group. Opposition or deviation from this societal norm was punishable by
execution, imprisonment, ostracism, or economic and political restraint.
This reality reinforced, and often dictated, a social style, which is often as-

sociated with prealcoholic personality traits (Segal, 1986). These traits include a high level of cultural or national dissonance, a mixture of passive aggressive behaviors toward authority figures, difficulties in interpersonal relationships, low self-esteem, and feelings of boredom, loneliness, and hopelessness.

Exploration of the origins of loneliness and despair among individuals, particularly in Russia, suggests that substance use is a coping mechanism to handle feelings of isolation and alienation. Because Soviet citizens were deprived of the freedom of expression and could not reveal their thoughts and opinions publicly, people created a double life. They shared their private thoughts in secret. As a result, double standards were established, no one was trusted, and the kitchen culture was created where a night in the kitchen (usually with a bottle of vodka) was the only safe place to discuss political issues and share one's personal problems (Kagan, 1992b).

Since the Soviets could not imagine expressing their feelings openly, they did not learn the skills necessary to do so. One had to appear cheerful and enthusiastic. One always had to demonstrate support and agreement with political and social issues, even if one genuinely disagreed with them. The Soviet system was always correct, and the capitalistic system, the enemy, was always viewed as "destructive, inhumane, and evil." This paranoid view of the world was promoted in education and in the media. Dr. Olga Marlin, a Czechoslovakian psychologist who now lives and works in New York City, says growing up in this kind of atmosphere can make people feel divided, guilty, and ashamed (Marlin, 1990). She further indicates that, in the totalitarian society, aggression was projected outside of the main group, to other individuals, groups, or systems (Marlin, 1994). There was a constant search for the external forces, or outside enemies, that were responsible for all the personal problems, misfortunes, and social and economic disadvantages of the nation and its individual citizens.

Since they have been taught to think only of the community, and not of themselves, most Russians drink in groups of three or more companions. The denial of independent thought and feeling is so strong that it is often only through intoxication that they can express their individuality.

Exploring the impact on the family is difficult. For example, as Soviet families feared for their safety, they drank vodka and secretly discussed and passed on to the next generation reports of executions and random arrests supported by the Communist regime. These private reports conflict with the international public portrayal of the people's commitment and loyalty to Mother Russia. This propaganda, promoted by the media, and the heartfelt loyalty Russians had for each other created a complex psychic and spiritual conflict. The picture of the Soviet Union that was conveyed to the Western world, with its abstract notions and simplistic black-and-white thinking, promoted an image of overwhelming submission and obedience, denial, abstractions from realistic thinking, and the suppression of emotions and personal expression. Ironically, Russians used to say, "We live only once, so drink and be happy." This informal slogan can be seen as a protest to the impersonal and hostile world where society itself can play the role of a cold, confused, and ambivalent parental figure (Kagan, 1996).

In the former Soviet Union, abusive interactions in families were culturally acceptable in most regions of the nation. There was an attitude of appropriateness, and even necessity, toward physical abuse by men of their wives and children. At home, males usually asserted their position of power with beatings. Alcoholic families in Russia were the very core of ongoing verbal abuse, emotional neglect, and domestic violence. When alcoholism has become an established phenomenon in the life of a family, there is usually little room for constructive communication. Alcohol abuse was an outlet for men who beat their wives to relieve themselves of responsibility for their actions (Gelles, 1974). Victims of family violence stay in the family unit in the hope that the periods between the fights will be longer and the periods of violence shorter. Thus, drunkenness can provide a time-out period when the norms of acceptable behaviors are disregarded (Grisham and Estes, 1986).

Political Views and Public Policies

Some hold the opinion that Soviet officials were somewhat against alcoholism and drug abuse but had tolerance for what Russians consider normal or casual drinking. What is considered casual drinking in Russia may be considered abusive by other standards. This tolerance toward drinking and substance abuse is viewed as a measure of social and political control of the population. It is likely that Soviet authorities took into account that a drunken society is not as likely to organize resistance efforts against a dictatorship as a sober one, and that, likewise, a drinking individual is easier to manipulate and control than a sober one (Segal, 1986).

Historically, narcological clinics in the former Soviet Union were designed to deal with late-stage alcoholics and focused exclusively on chronic alcoholism. Treatment models, which emphasized a biomedical model of addiction, lacked the financial backing to address the national problem of drinking alcohol. Since the collapse of the Soviet Union, the abuse of other drugs has reached epidemic proportions. Narcological clinics have not been prepared for the epidemic of drug and alcohol abuse.

As in other developing nations, treatment and prevention efforts were not a priority among the health concerns of the central government in the former Soviet Union. Considering the fact that the use of alcohol and other drugs is dramatically increasing, prevention and intervention strategies are urgently needed. The prohibitive legislative attempts to control drug and alcohol use are not sufficient to address a national drinking problem. It is well documented, internationally, that punitive, legal, and medical approaches alone do not adequately address substance-abuse issues. For example, the attempt of the Soviet government to curtail the sale of vodka by controlling per capita sales in 1985 was similar to the attempt made at prohibition in the United States; both failed.

During this period, administrative measures were established to control purchases per person, as well as hours of operation for liquor vendors. Sobering-up stations were set up in the community but often involved a criminal penalty for people identified as alcoholic. These punitive approaches exacerbated the problem; illegal alcohol production increased sharply, 40 percent of the *samogon* was being made in the cities, and the number of closet substance abusers increased proportionately.

The ineffectiveness of prohibition efforts, and the lack of recognition and disregard of the social, psychological, and medical services needed to address substance-abuse problems, has driven the problem from the mainstream to the underground. In the former Soviet Union, alcoholism was not viewed as a family disease, but as a state disease (Kagan, 1996).

THE FUTURE OF SUBSTANCE ABUSE IN RUSSIA

Russian clinicians have embraced the disease concept and the medical model of addiction treatment. The traditional Russian model, which maintains a narrow focus on the substance abuser, consists of detoxification, drug therapy to alleviate withdrawal symptoms, hypnosis or recoding against substance use, aversive therapy, and Pavlovian behavior modification. Treatment efforts included sobering-up stations, a unique Soviet creation for fast detoxification; social humiliation; and in some cases, branding the individual as an alcoholic. Confidentiality for addicts is a concept unfamiliar to clinicians in the CIS.

Alternative, or modern, substance-abuse treatment approaches used in Russia include the use of herbal remedies, often associated with folk medicine; hypnosis or coding; and breath work (Shafer, 1994). Dr. Drosdov, director of Narcology No. 17 (the largest substance-abuse treatment center in Moscow), states that the treatment methods at his facility include special methods to arouse the patient's disgust for alcohol. These techniques include the use of a biological method called "sparing therapy," which is based on the use of amino acids. It is claimed that it has no side effects.

Dr. Balashov, a clinical director of the Adolescent Unit at the same center, described the Russian medical model as quite sophisticated. Practitioners, however, lack the knowledge and understanding of the social and psychological aspects of the disease common among practitioners in the West (from an interview with Dr. Balashov, 1992). Additionally, there is a lack of knowledge about enabling and codependency, terms often associated with the family's response to substance-abusing members. Therefore, Russian professionals tend to view the family members of the substance abuser as suffering victims of substance abuse, not as having a role in the addiction or recovery processes. Alcoholism, in particular, is seen as an unfortunate part of most Russian families, an element that needs to be survived by the non-alcoholic family members.

As a result of years of poor diet and medical care, in the CIS and Soviet Union, by the time a person reaches the late stages of addiction, he has serious medical problems. Such problems often require expensive prescribed medications, which patients cannot afford, and often results in abuse and dependency on the prescribed drugs, or illicit street drugs from the underground and Mafia.

Attitudes toward addicts by health-care staff are often unfriendly and negative. Therefore, Russian clients do not express an interest and willingness to participate in therapy, especially substance-abuse counseling. They fear being stigmatized, labeled, and punished by the agencies they turn to for help. Most of all, they fear that exposing their substance-abuse problems can affect their status (Kagan, 1997a).

Programs offering social and psychological rehabilitation are extremely limited. Medical facilities vary in their approaches to treatment. Most interventions, unlike treatment in the West and the United States, are based on pharmacotherapy. Russian drug treatment involves virtually no individual psychotherapy, group therapy, or education that addresses the addict's thoughts of overcoming addiction (Shafer, 1994).

Traditional treatment methods based on self-disclosure, trust, and group support appear to be culturally inappropriate for Russian substance abusers (Kagan and Shafer, 2001). The concept of confidentiality is viewed with skepticism and misunderstanding. For example, it is not unusual for a client to say, "I know this is confidential, you explained that to me, but please, don't share what I am about to tell you with anyone." This issue became evident during a training program for clinicians in Kiev, Ukraine, and in Saint Petersburg, Russia (Shafer, 1994). Former Soviets are accustomed to having their privacy violated by the KGB and by other authority figures. The former Soviet citizen, seeking help, struggles with trusting the health-care professional.

In treatment, it usually takes time and great skill to establish a rapport with Russian substance abusers. They expect a double message similar to the one they received from the Soviet government. Soviets fear that everything will be reported to the government. This fear of revealing personal information upon request, especially to officials or persons perceived to be in authority, has valid historical roots (Kagan and Shafer, 2001).

After the October Revolution in 1917, alcoholics were registered with the government as soon as they were caught by the militia (police) and were sent to sobering-up stations. During the Bolshevik regime, the word "alcoholic" or "drug-addict" was stamped onto the person's domestic passport. After his visit to the sobering-up station, everyone within the person's social circle was informed about the incident. Additionally, the family was made responsible to pay for the involuntary detoxification, and a severe warning was sent to his or her employer (Shafer, 1994).

When a person carries an official label of alcoholic, it is easy to understand the difficulty of entering a formal treatment setting. In this atmosphere, imagine attending an AA meeting and sharing feelings in front of strangers (Kagan and Shafer, 2001). Dr. J.W. Yandow (1992) and Dr. K. Shafer (1994) noted, after visiting state psychiatric and narcological hospitals in the former USSR, that schizophrenia and alcoholism were diagnoses given to political dissidents, who were then heavily medicated and guarded by the Russian military and police dogs at treatment facilities.

CONCLUSION

The earlier period of the Communist government and reorganization of the Soviet Union created a culture prone to alcoholism and substance use. The continuously changing political and economic climate has made life extremely difficult and, as a result, has encouraged alcohol and drug abuse as an escape measure.

According to Segal (2000), societal changes, such as urbanization, migration, social disorganization, political unrest, and loss of community support, have set the stage for increases in excessive drinking and substance use. Rapid acculturation can increase maladjustment when the exposure to change is greater than the desire for change. Rapid acceptance of values and belief systems from massive tourism and exposure to media from other countries can increase the separation from the group of origin and thus weaken the support and reliance from primary support groups (Kagan and Shafer, 2001). Despite the fact that the majority of Russians are highly educated and sophisticated, they are unprepared for the absence of ordinary services, such as socialized housing, child care, employment, and free medical and dental care provided in the Soviet system. Moreover, Russians tend to be extremely resistant to using traditional mental health services, owing to confidentiality issues and fears of exposure, and they can be inappropriately demanding of certain medical services that in the past were readily available to them. The majority of Russians are not ready to recognize various mental-health and substance-abuse problems as being significant and as requiring special consideration and treatment.

There are a number of concerns that seem specific to Soviets and now to Russian CIS citizens. These concerns are particularly associated with excessive drinking, drug abuse, and domestic violence. Since the Russian culture is viewed as endorsing heavy drinking, specifically vodka, it seems logical to apply the biopsychosocial and spiritual models of assessing substance-abuse problems. The pressures of cultural fragmentation, mistrust of authority figures, family problems, and migration of people in and out of this formerly closed-off society all compound the treatment issues of the Russian substance user.

Communication and the opening of the Soviet borders will provide much needed information. Never before have clinicians in this part of the world had the opportunity for international collaboration, nor have they had the ability to explore Western methods of addiction treatment (Shafer, 1994).

REFERENCES

Anderson, D.J. (1992, August 4). Hazelden report: Russia hopes to adapt western treatment methods. *Star Tribune* (Minneapolis, MN), p. 8E.

Bureau of European Affairs. (2000, May). *Background Notes: Russia*. Washington, D.C.: U.S. Department of State.

Davis, R.B. (1994). Drug and alcohol use in the former Soviet Union. *International Journal of the Addictions, 19 (3)*, 303–309.

Dover, E. (1992). Personal communication. Interview with Dr. E. Drozdov, head physician at Moscow's Narcological Hospital No. 17.

Gelles, R.J. (1974). *The violent home: A study of physical aggression between husbands and wives*. Beverly Hills, CA: Sage Publications.

Grisham, K.J., & Estes, N.J. (1986). Dynamics of alcoholic families. In *Alcoholism: Development, consequences, and interventions* (3rd ed.) (pp. 303–316). St. Louis, MO: C.V. Mosby.

Kagan, H. (1992a, September) *America and Russia: Recovery options at work*. Paper presented at the Sixth Annual Great Lakes Conference on Addictions, Indianapolis, IN.

———. (1992b, October). *Improving refugee access to mental health and substance abuse services*. Paper presented at the African/Russian Refugee Conference, Denver, CO.

———. (1994, October). *Russian emigre's maladjustment and substance abuse as a social problem*. Paper presented at the National Conference on Refugee Resettlement, Washington, DC.

———. (1995–1996). Alcoholism and physical abusive interactions between adult parents and their children. *Jewish Board of Family and Children Services: Grand Rounds, 3*. New York: Kellner/McCaffrey.

———. (1996). *Between two worlds: Understanding emigre mental health needs*. Paper presented at the UJA (United Jewish Appeal) Federation, New York.

———. (1997a, May). *The unique experience of the family oriented treatment program for Russian substance abusers*. Paper presented at the 29th annual NASW (National Association of Social Work) Alcoholism Institute, New York.

———. (1997b, August). *Women, ethnicity & substance abuse: Irish, African & Russian-American perspectives*. Paper presented at the "Matinee on Broadway," Liberty Management Group, New York.

Kagan, H. and Shafer, K. (2001). *Russian-speaking substance abusers in transition: New country, old problems*. In Shulamith, L. and Ashenberg, S. (Eds.), *Ethnocultural factors in substance abuse treatment*. New York: Guilford Press.

Kissin, M. (1991, December). *Culturally sensitive interviewing in the psychological assessment of Russian refugees.* Paper presented at the National Conference on Health and Mental Health of Soviet Refugees, Chicago, IL.

Landau, J. (1982). Therapy with families in cultural transition. In M. McGoldric, J.K. Pierce, and J. Giordono (Eds.), *Ethnicity and family therapy* (pp. 552–572). New York: Guilford Press.

Marlin, O. (1990, Spring). Group psychology in the totalitarian system: A psychoanalytic view. *Group*, pp. 44–58.

———. (1994). Special issues in the analytic treatment of immigrants and refugees. *Issues in Psychoanalytic Psychology, 16* (1), 7–16.

McRae, H. (1997). The strange case of falling birth rates in the West. Infonautics Corporation. Retrieved July 25, 2000, from the World Wide Web: http://www.infonautics.com.

Paredes, A. (1986). Models and definitions of alcoholism. In *Alcoholism: Development, consequences, and interventions* (3rd ed.) (pp. 53–66). St. Louis, MO: C.V. Mosby.

Segal, B.M. (1986). The Soviet heavy-drinking culture and the American heavy-drinking subculture. *Alcohol and Culture: Comparative Perspectives from Europe and America* (pp. 149–160). New York: New York Academy of Sciences.

———. (1987). *Russian drinking: Use and abuse of alcohol in pre-revolutionary Russia.* New Brunswick, NJ: Rutgers Center of Alcohol Studies.

———. (1990). *The drunken society: Alcohol abuse and alcoholism in the Soviet Union.* New York: Hippocrene Books.

———. (December 16, 2000). Author's Personal communication about the current status of substance abuse in Russia.

Shafer, K. (1994). A study of the effectiveness of alcohol and drug abuse training for professionals in Russia and the Ukraine. *Dissertation Abstracts International.*

Specter, M. (1997, November 4). At a western outpost of Russia, AIDS spreads "like a forest fire." *New York Times*, pp. A1, A10.

Traynor, I. (2000, June 30). Russia dying of drink and despair. England: Guardian Unlimited, Guardian Newspapers Limited.

Wines, M. (2000, April 26). Zhdanovo Journal. Intoxicated With Religion (and Quite Literally) *New York Times*, p. A1.

Wright, M.K. (1994, Fall). Russians learn about western approach to addiction. *Treatment Today*, pp. 11–13.

Yandow, V.W. (1992, November–December). Substance abuse treatment in Russia and Hungary. *Addiction & Recovery*, pp. 42–45.

12

SWITZERLAND

Andrew Cherry

INTRODUCTION

Switzerland adopted a harm-reduction model for drug-abuse control, although Switzerland's progress in this area has not been watched as closely as that in the Netherlands. The Swiss moved ahead with drug policies favoring reduced penalties for drug use, and toward drug legalization. Perhaps because the focus of the U.S. antidrug war was not on Switzerland, that small country was able to develop strategies to reduce the harm caused by drugs sold to Swiss citizens by the global, illegal drug cartels.

The Swiss model shows serious flaws in the prohibition model's ability to manage the harm from illegal drug consumption. After a serious outbreak in addiction in Switzerland in the 1980s, the Swiss began to explore and adopt diverse drug policies in part based on the harm-reduction model. These policies led to a reduction in penalties for drug use and, in the 1994 experimental program, the provision of medically prescribed narcotics (primarily heroin) to registered addicts. To determine whether an individual was an addict and needed to receive medically prescribed heroin, the addict had to be over 20 years of age, have been using illegal drugs for the past two years, and had to show signs of deterioration in health or social functioning (Satel and Aeschbach, 1999).

After a period of service, a program evaluation was conducted to determine the effectiveness of the program on criminal involvement among the participants. Several measures were used to determine the participants' continued involvement in crime while they were using prescription heroin. Records of convictions, police records, extensive interviews (conducted every six months), and instruments measuring self-reported delinquency and victimization were used as data to describe the behavior of the addicted participants. The results of the study showed substantial drops in the prevalence and incidence of misdemeanors and more serious crime, as well as in victimization among participants in the prescription heroin program. The study also found that, in retrospect, delinquency and victimization among this group of addicts were closely correlated with becoming addicted to heroin (Satel and Aeschbach, 1999).

Heroin addiction is a serious problem in Switzerland, and there was concern that a program giving away free heroin would increase the percentage of people who would try heroin. About 1.3 percent of Swiss between the ages of fifteen and thirty-nine had used heroin or methadone at least once in 1992, and that percentage (1.4 percent) remained relatively the same in 1997. Although having nothing whatsoever to do with the heroin program, the use of marijuana and hashish increased from 16.3 percent in 1992 to 26.7 percent in 1997. There was also an increase in cocaine and stimulants use from 3.8 percent in 1992 to 5.8 percent in 1997 (see Table 12.1) (Swiss Federal Office of Public Health, 1999).

While cannabis use increased in the 1990s, alcohol consumption in Switzerland declined during the same period. This decline may have long-term effects. In 2000 officials estimated that between 2,500 and 3,500 Swiss die each year from excessive alcohol consumption. Although per capita alcohol consumption has declined from 10.1 liters (10.67 quarts) per person to 9.2 liters (9.7 quarts), it is still high when compared to other European nations, with the exception of France. In France, alcohol consumption was 17 liters (17.96 quarts) per person at the end of the 1990s (Institute of Alcohol Studies, 1997; Swiss Alcohol Board, 2000).

A Brief Profile of Switzerland

The Swiss typically refer to their country as Confoederatio Helvetica; therefore, the abbreviation often associated with Switzerland is CH. The cross and the colors of the Swiss flag have a religious origin: The white cross is a symbol for the cross on which Jesus was crucified, and the red color surrounding the cross represents the blood of Christ. The official languages of Switzerland are German, French, Italian, and Romantsch (the language of the indigenous people). However, official documents and declarations need only be in German, French, and Italian (Hilowitz, 1990).

Switzerland's independence and neutrality have long been honored by the major European powers. It was neutral through both World War I (1914–1918) and World War II (1939–1945). Although the country refused to join the United Nations (UN), the political and economic integration of Europe over the last half of the twentieth century, as well as Switzerland's

Table 12.1
Changes in Drug Use Over Time among the Swiss between the Ages of
Fifteen and Thirty-nine

Types of Drugs	1992	1997
Hashish/Marijuana	16.3%	26.7%
Cocaine/Stimulants	3.8%	5.8%
Heroin/Methadone	1.3%	1.4%

Source: Swiss Federal Office of Public Health, 1999.

role in many UN and international organizations, may be overshadowing the country's concern for its neutrality. Switzerland is not quite twice the size of New Jersey. It has a population of slightly over seven million people (7,262,372 estimated in mid-2000). Three major ethnic groups make up the Swiss population: German, 65 percent; French, 18 percent; and Italian, 10 percent. Others include Romansch, 1 percent; and other, 6 percent. In 1990 religious preferences included Roman Catholic, 46.1 percent; Protestant, 40 percent; other, 5 percent; and none, 8.9 percent, (Hilowitz, 1990).

Switzerland, a landlocked nation, is the crossroads between Northern and Southern Europe. Switzerland shares her borders with Austria, France, Italy, Liechtenstein, and Germany. Primarily a mountainous country, it contains some of the highest mountains in Europe (Alps in the south, Jura in the northwest). The remainder of the country is made up of a central plateau of rolling hills, plains, and large lakes.

The social indicators are very positive in Switzerland; it has one of the highest standards of living in the world. Infant mortality rates are 4.53 deaths per 1,000 live births (2000 estimate). Life expectancy at birth in the year 2000 was 79.6 years for the total population: 76.73 years for males and 82.63 years for females (2000 estimates). The unemployment rate was 1.7 percent in September 2000. The GPA per person was $35,500 (U.S.) (Australia Department of Foreign Affairs and Trade, 2000).

Switzerland has a well-developed, industrialized economy based on watches and precision instruments. Switzerland is also a major international financial center. Financiers from around the world have Swiss accounts because of the stability of Swiss banks and the traditional secrecy regarding banking transactions.

Switzerland's neutrality has always been a bit mystifying given its small size and its location surrounded by much larger countries. Switzerland became a neutral country only after many years of being controlled by the Romans, Germanic tribes, the Franks, the Germans a second time, and the

Holy Roman Empire. The Swiss cantons (or states) organized a mutual defense league in 1291 after the Holy Roman Empire tried to claim feudal control of Switzerland. After more than 200 years of Swiss resistance, Holy Roman Emperor Maximilian I was defeated in 1499. The Treaty of Basel required the empire to recognize the independence of Switzerland. Three hundred years later, in 1798, the French, under Napoléon Bonaparte's rule, established the Helvetic Republic. The French military occupation was offensive to many Swiss. After Napoléon's defeat, the Congress of Vienna (1815) recognized the neutrality of Switzerland.

A number of large international organizations are located in Switzerland. The country actively participates in several worldwide and European trade organizations. In 1992, however, Swiss voters rejected a proposal to participate in a European free-trade zone. In many ways this vote confirmed the Swiss desire to maintain Switzerland's distinctive characteristic of international neutrality (Hilowitz, 1990).

VIGNETTE

Friedrick was not feeling well as he made his way to the injection room near a local hospital. He felt like he was coming down with a cold. He entered the room in the back of the clinic, a well-lit room with several sterile medical tables surrounded by comfortable chairs and couches, the kind used in waiting rooms and lobbies. Each table held a candle and a kidney-shaped dish. Inside the dish was a sterile syringe, a spoon, a small vial of sterile water, a rubber tourniquet, cotton, and a Band-Aid. Mirrors line the walls for addicts who must inject the heroin in a neck vein because the veins in their arms, legs, and groin have collapsed.

The nurse greeted Friedrick as he approached her desk. While he was signing in, he told her that he thought he was catching a cold. She asked him about his most recent drug use to determine whether it was a drug-related lung infection. She took him into an examining room where she gave him a physical. She checked his tattered arms and legs for infected veins often caused by injecting drugs with unclean needles. After determining he was probably suffering from a common cold, she gave him advice on how to reduce the risk of his heroin use aggravating his cold and turning the cold into pneumonia. After he dressed, he made his payment and went over to one of the sterile tables and sat down. As the nurse stood by, in case she was needed to provide instruction in the proper injection of heroin in a particular part of the body, or to intervene in the case of an overdose, Friedrick prepared the single dose of heroin, took off his left shoe and sock, and injected himself in a vein between his toes. Friedrick had become an expert at finding a vein that could still take an injection. Often, the new nurses at the injection room had stared at him in amazement as he eased the needle in a vein that had not been visible moments before. He and the nurse were both a bit mesmerized as they watched the red blood he drew up into the plastic syringe swirl mysteriously in the clear liquid heroin inside the plunger. After he injected himself, as if in slow motion, he set the syringe in the bowl on the table and put the cotton alcohol swab between his toes to stop any bleeding. After a short period, when he did not move, Friedrick got up and fixed himself a cup of coffee. About ten minutes later, Friedrick said to the nurse, "I feel better. I'll see you later." And he left. Friedrick returned to his safe-injection room several times that day to receive his high-quality individualized dose of heroin. The cost of his daily habit was only a fraction of what it would cost on the street, but the cost still kept him running from one job to another, even when he did not feel like it.

OVERVIEW OF SUBSTANCE ABUSE IN SWITZERLAND AND BASIC DEMOGRAPHICS

Switzerland is neither a member of the European Union, nor a member of the United Nations. Even so, Switzerland is a signatory of the UN Single Convention Treaty on Narcotic Drugs (1961). The treaty was signed only after specific provisions were written in for the Swiss. These provisions included the right to continue to grow cannabis as a farm crop. After the treaty was signed, nothing changed on the Swiss drug scene until the late 1970s; then the global wave of drug use among the young, particularly in the United States, exploded and, in time, began to impact the youth of Europe. In response, the Swiss government took a hard-line position on all drug use, especially heroin. A convicted heroin dealer could be imprisoned for as many as twenty years. Like prohibition efforts before and since, the new hard line against heroin resulted in a higher incidence of heroin experimentation and abuse. As the 1980s drew to a close, heroin use and abuse among the young in Switzerland was out of control. During this period, the People's Park in Zurich became an asylum for heroin users, and the park became known as "Needle Park" (Klingemann, 1996).

By the end of the 1980s, the Swiss had realized that using the criminal justice system to control drug use was not working. The police arrested the heroin users, who often turned out to be the children of their neighbors and friends. Officials also realized that, if the drug users were not kept in prison, they would continue to use drugs. They would also continue to be exposed to unregulated heroin, heroin dealers, and criminals who traffic in heroin; and they had access to other drugs and contraband. In 1989 the Swiss Narcotics Commission, after considering several drug-control models, selected a harm-reduction public-health model to control drug use and abuse. Based on this model and on the experiences of other countries, the commission recommended a more tolerant approach, even advocating the legalization of personal possession and the use of all substances (Olson, 1998).

Although, at the beginning of the twenty-first century, drugs for personal use were illegal in Switzerland, a number of initiatives and policies had been approved and implemented to provide heroin users with sterilized needles. Injection rooms, where heroin users could inject themselves safely, were opened in some Swiss states. In October 1997, the Swiss people overwhelmingly supported continuing a humane and tolerant policy toward heroin users; 71 percent voted against a referendum that would have ended tolerant methods of dealing with heroin use (Olson, 1998).

HISTORY OF ALCOHOL AND DRUG ABUSE IN SWITZERLAND

Illegal drug use in Switzerland does not have much of a history. The first legislation of any kind related to illicit drugs in Switzerland dates back to 1924, when the government gave in to pressure from the United States to sign international treaties to fight illegal drugs on a global scale. However, in the 1960s, drugs did become an issue for the Swiss. Before the 1970s, drug use was a personal choice that was not questioned unless it created problems for the drug user, his family, or the community. The hippie movement changed that view for many in Switzerland as it did in many other countries. In 1969 around 500 people were arrested for some form of cannabis offense. Only a very small number were arrested for an opiate offense. The first registered illicit-drug-related death occurred in the city of Zurich in 1972; very few cocaine cases showed up in 1974. The second revision of the national illicit drug laws took place in 1975. This policy took a hard-line stance against drug use. The following years saw a steady rise in the number of drug users and of drug traffickers, and many came to believe that the increase was caused by the policing approach to the control of drug use (Klingemann, 1996).

Zurich's Needle Park

To get to the infamous Needle Park in Zurich, one passes by streets lined with Swiss and international banks in Switzerland's financial district. The park is located behind the National Museum of Switzerland.

By 1986 the drug scene in the city of Zurich, which came to symbolize the Swiss attitude toward drug use, settled in the Platzspitz (Needle Park). It was estimated that, at the height of the drug epidemic, there were 3,000 heroin users in the Zurich area. It was an open drug market. The conditions in the park were unsanitary, and needle sharing was rampant. As blood-borne diseases increased, the health of the drug users deteriorated. By 1992 the mortality rates from drug overdoses had tripled. At that point, public tolerance was exhausted, and the police closed the Platzspitz. Decentralization of treatment, and coercion for the addict to participate in treatment, became the new approach. However, because of the AIDS threat, drug pol-icy shifted to a harm-reduction approach (Farrell and Hall, 1998; Satel and Aeschbach, 1999).

In many ways, the heroin drug scene in Needle Park was a public service. It was a truth that supported the rational argument that addiction was a festering wound in the body of society. Seeing that human tragedy in the pastoral setting of a city park somehow changed forever the view that a heroin addiction was "cool." The scene of people sitting around a park bench "firing up" and shooting themselves with heroin they drew from a smutty, bent spoon assaulted our consciousness and insulted us with the gory details of the enormous number of lives wasted by drugs. It is clear why most cities try to hide the problem, or attempt to chase it away.

The Discovery of LSD

In many ways, the discovery of lysergic acid diethylamide (LSD) was the start of the "brave new world." The designer drugs that followed were a series of "moods on tap." These drugs, unlike drugs used as medication, were never meant to cure a physical illness. These drugs were designed to allow the user to predetermine the mood he or she wished to experience. Probably the most interesting characteristic of such drugs is their ability to mimic moods that in the past had always seemed to occur without inside stimulation. It was always thought that something caused the anger, passion, aggression, exhilaration, paranoia, fearlessness, discovery, etc., but no one knew what. Designer drugs changed all that. If you wish to be happy, take Ecstasy; if you want to be numb, overdose on benzodiazepines; if you want to be king of the world, take an amphetamine; if you want the insight of a mystic, take LSD (Huxley, 1954).

During World War II, a Basle chemist, Dr. Albert Hofmann, ingested a minute quantity of an ergot derivative (four-millionths of a gram), and a whole new world opened up to humankind. Ergot is a wheat blight, a fun-gus that kills the wheat plant before it matures. It had been used to ease childbirth for many years. Hofmann was trying to develop a synthetic ergot because collecting ergot from Swiss wheat fields was laborious and produced limited supplies. There are special fields in small Swiss mountain valleys where wheat blight is allowed to live so it will infect the wheat plants, and the infected plants can be gathered and used to make medications.

This minute amount of ergot derivative (LSD) taken by Hofmann was not expected to do much. However, while he was cycling home with his assistant, he began to have strange symptoms. "My field of vision swayed before me and was distorted like the reflections in an amusement park mir-ror. I had the impression of being unable to move from the spot, although my assistant later told me that we had cycled at a good pace." He also reported other startling symptoms: vertigo and visual disturbances ("the faces of those around me appeared as grotesque, colored masks"). He reported marked motor activity that alternated with paralysis. At times, he remembered feeling that his head, limbs, and entire body were filled with lead. He reported a dry, constricted sensation in his throat. He had a clear recognition that he sometimes observed, in the manner of an independent, neutral observer, his behavior at a distance. Occasionally he reported feeling as if he were out of his body (Strassman, 1995).

In the mid-1940s, there was a great deal of interest in investigating new drugs that might be capable of causing unique moods and changing other types of human behavior. In some groups, like the Central Intelligence Agency (CIA), the interest in LSD was due to the hope that the visions induced by the drug could be used to brainwash individuals or be used in combat to disorient enemy forces. In another area of science, because the visions produced by LSD resemble those reported by psychotic patients, a few psychiatrists at the time, such as Humphrey Osmond, began experimenting with LSD in the hope it might help in the treatment of schizophrenia and other mental disorders. The reaction of any one individual, however, could not be consistently predicted. The reports outside of the CIA of fantastic personal insights of those who used LSD intrigued both the philosopher and the psychiatrist. Vision-inducing drugs, such as LSD, mescaline, peyote, psilocybin mushrooms, tobacco (nicotine is a psychedelic), and morning glory seeds, would have remained dormant for many more years if Humphrey Osmond had not convinced Aldous Huxley to take a trip on mescaline (Huxley, 1954).

Following the publication of Aldous Huxley's *The Doors of Perception* in 1954, there was a slow resurgence of interest in vision-inducing drugs. The young, who were disillusioned with U.S. materialism and later militarism, were more willing by the 1960s to listen to Huxley's argument for trying LSD. He suggested that a drug such as LSD would heighten or alter one's perceptions and was worth enjoying, not just in its own right, but also for the new insights and the new meanings it could provide.

I am not so foolish as to equate what happens under the influence of mescaline or of any other drug, prepared or in the future preparable, with the realization of the end and ultimate purpose of human life. All I am suggesting is that the mescaline experience is what Catholic theologians call "a gratuitous grace," not necessary for salvation, but potentially helpful and to be accepted thankfully, if made available. To be shaken out of the ruts of ordinary perception, to be shown for a few timeless hours the outer and the inner world, not as they appear to an animal obsessed with survival or to a human being obsessed with words and notions, but as they are apprehended, directly and unconditionally, by Mind at Large—this is an experience of inestimable value to everyone and especially to the intellectual. (Huxley, 1954, p. 73)

A problem arose, however, for those who were foolish enough, or overwhelmingly curious, or determined to seek insight; mescaline was difficult to find. The raw material, peyote, is scarce and found only in the southwestern desert area of the United States. It was used by the North American Plains Indians in religious rituals for at least a thousand years, but they had never needed much. At the time, thousands and eventually millions of people around the world took a vision-inducing drug.

Albert Hofmann's LSD was the answer. It produced a mental state similar to that of mescaline, and LSD could be manufactured in a laboratory. LSD quickly became the standard drug for those seeking the mystic experience. Moreover, scientific trials confirmed the experience reported by earlier users. These were mental experiences that "enhanced values or expanded the self, a road to love and better relationships, a device for art appreciation, or a spur to creative endeavors, a means of insight, and a door to religious experience." This was great for the majority, but the consequence of taking LSD for a few individuals was a "bad trip"—experiences that were highly disturbing and often terrifying, such as sensations of dying from an overdose (Strassman, 1995).

The formula for LSD was well known; the materials to make LSD were available; the chemistry lab in many high schools and every college in the United States had the equipment to manufacture LSD. In addition to being tasteless, odorless, and colorless, LSD was not bulky. It was easy to transport and sell in small amounts in the form of tablets. Once more, legal prohibitions were employed in an attempt to stop young people from using LSD. Prohibition was immediately followed by an increase in the availability of LSD and by an increase in the demand (Brecher, 1972). The increased availability should have been explained in part by the higher prices caused by law enforcement arrests and drug busts to confiscate LSD. The higher prices attracted more people to deal in LSD. The increased demand can similarly be explained in part by the publicity LSD received during periods when legislative action was taken against it. As in the case of opiates, barbiturates, amphetamines, glue, and other drugs, the public warnings became a public announcement of the availability of a new drug, and this publicity was a lure to the disenfranchised youth.

The psychedelic movement eventually split into two main groups based on the views of Humphrey Osmond. He suggested that psychedelic drugs (a name he coined to describe vision-inducing drugs) "provide a chance, perhaps only a slender one, for homo faber, the cunning, ruthless, foolhardy pleasure-greedy toolmaker, to merge into that other creature whose presence we have so rashly presumed, homo sapiens the wise, the understanding, the compassionate" (Inglis, 1975; p. 215). Some of Osmond's followers took this to mean that the drug was simply to reveal, to anybody who took it, the limitations he had been imposing on himself; so that he would seek ways, not necessarily through drugs, to explore the potential within himself which he had not known existed. Others, including Dr. Timothy Leary, promoted LSD as having almost magical powers. By the mid-1970s, the Leary version of the role of LSD in society, "turn on, tune in, and drop out," which resulted in millions of U.S. young people taking LSD, was going out of fashion. Tripping on LSD became a novel experience that a few adolescents tried in their late teens, but as a movement, it dissipated. The LSD movement was more of a fad. After an individual used LSD once or several times, there was nowhere to go with the movement. The thought was that LSD would help us better understand ourselves, and if we could accept ourselves, we could learn to love others. "Tripping" on LSD as a way to improve society was not a good fit within that society at the time, and the movement died out (Strassman, 1995).

Toward the end of his psychiatric career, Osmond was clear in what psychedelics, visionary drugs such as mescaline, and LSD had done for the understanding of the human mind. For the first time in psychiatry, there was no dispute that when a mental patient said he or she experienced a hallucination, he or she did see it and it was as real as anything anyone reports seeing and feeling. Osmond was also able to classify an additional set of human conditions that will produce similar visions: high fever, sleep deprivation, and extreme hunger. Humphrey Osmond finished his training as a psychiatrist in Austria and met Albert Hofmann after reading the report of Hofmann's experience with LSD. Later, in Canada's midwest, he took mescaline during a religious ritual in an American Indian village and found the experience miraculous. Later, he guided Huxley though the experience that resulted in the book *The Doors of Perception*.

Osmond contributed a great deal to the treatment of mental illness. He came up with the idea of vitamin therapy for schizophrenia in the early 1950s and, at the time, his vitamin therapy worked better than most drug therapies. He also corresponded with Carl Jung who disclosed to Osmond that he had experienced many years of paranoia in his early adulthood. Jung also told Osmond that in many ways LSD was not like insanity. Insanity, Jung said, came on so subtly that the victim does not even realize it has occurred.

At a mental hospital where severe drug addicts were being treated, one young schizophrenic said he had tried every illegal drug available. He reported that the only drug that reminded him of schizophrenia was an overdose on amphetamines or cocaine (Osmond, 1977).

Osmond's only regret, at the end of his career, was that the U.S. government and other funders in the mid-1960s stopped funding all research of LSD. Osmond still believed that psychedelics could be useful in the treatment of severe alcoholism and drug addiction and in other emotional disorders that are treated with insight therapy (Osmond, 1977).

THE SUBSTANCE ABUSE PROBLEM IN SWITZERLAND TODAY

Political Views and Public Policies

Another way of looking at the political and social agreement in Switzerland is to review their national votes on liberalizing their drug laws. Two major votes in 1997 and 1998 set the course for Switzerland.

In 1997 an overwhelming majority of 70 percent of voters rejected the Youth without Drugs initiative, which called for full abstinence. The issue was put to a national referendum after the right-of-center Swiss People's Party collected 140,000 signatures in support of the proposal. The national referendum proposed to introduce a hard-line, antidrug policy. Sponsors of the Youth without Drugs referendum believed that the government's anti-drug policy was sending the wrong signal and, in effect, encouraged Swiss youth to experiment with drugs. To this group of Swiss, the government's distribution of heroin was the equivalent of a distorted form of legal death. On the other side of this referendum were mainstream church groups, trade unions, the police, the vast majority of youth, and those working with the addicted. The vast majority of Swiss said, in effect, that the government's harm-reduction programs should continue uninterrupted. This vote also supported the continuation of the program to provide hard-core heroin addicts, who had been unable to maintain recovery after trying all forms of alternative therapies, with medically prescribed heroin. These programs also offered addicts methadone and other heroin substitutes in an effort to keep heroin addicts from buying illegal drugs (Olson, 1998).

In 1998 Swiss voters were asked once again to vote on the illegal drug issue. In this case, the referendum asked voters to approve decriminalizing "the consumption, cultivation or possession of drugs, and their acquisition for personal use." This referendum was no less controversial than the 1997 referendum. None of the main political parties actively supported the campaign, and the government was appalled at the prospect of becoming a supplier and distributor of hard and soft drugs. Government officials warned that a "yes" vote could turn Switzerland into a "paradise for the Mafia" and a magnet for "drug tourists" who would be attracted by readily available soft and hard drugs (Olson, 1998).

Proponents of the drug-legalization referendum, led by a group of socialists and medical doctors, argued that legalizing drugs would break the back of Switzerland's flourishing black market in drugs. It would also save the country hundreds of millions of dollars in the time spent on law enforcement.

A leading Swiss magazine, *L'Illustre*, in a national poll conducted at the time, reported that among those polled who opposed legalization of all drugs, 40 percent were willing to back the legal sale of marijuana to people over eighteen years of age. Additionally, over 50 percent supported the sale of marijuana for medical purposes (Shields, 1998).

Many Swiss officials feared that drug liberalization would nullify their efforts to deal with Switzerland's serious problem with drugs. Based on statistics from the European Monitoring Center for Drugs and Drug Addiction in Lisbon, Portugal, they made the point that drug use in Switzerland was among the highest in Europe. Drug use in Switzerland per 1,000 adults was exceeded only by Italy, Spain, and Luxembourg. One other fear of the officials was that Switzerland would end up isolated from other drug-fighting nations, and it was believed that, without partners to help fight the drug problem at the international level, international criminals and money laundering would increase in Switzerland.

The proponents for legalization pointed out that as fewer and fewer drug users were prosecuted and programs were set up to provide heroin and heroin substitutes to addicts, the number of new drug users in Switzerland actually went down. It was a reaction of the young to reality. When heroin addicts began picking up medical heroin at the drugstore (like other mental health patients), heroin lost its appeal as the ultimate "rebel drug," and heroin addiction was viewed as a drug used by pathetic addicts. In large part, because of these programs to dispense heroin, the number of heroin addicts held steady throughout the 1990s at a rate of roughly 30,000 addicts (Farrell and Hall, 1998).

Proponents also pointed out that the number of addicts in treatment went up, and the death from drug overdoses went down. Also important for the average Swiss citizen, addict-related crime and new HIV cases decreased markedly after the heroin program was instituted. The implication was that, by legally dispensing drugs, the same positive effect on areas where there were still problems, such as separating hard-drug sellers and soft-drug users, could be accomplished. The object of this model is to separate supply systems. When supply systems are separated, there is no need for soft-drug users to come into contact with the criminal element who, while selling marijuana or other soft drugs, also sell cocaine, heroin, guns, women and children, and other contraband.

Both sides had good arguments, but the Swiss public wanted a middle-of-the-road policy. Accordingly, 75 percent rejected the idea of legalizing all drugs. At the end of the twentieth century, the citizenry of Switzerland was not yet ready to legalize both hard and soft drugs. They also were not ready to go back to a criminal justice system approach for dealing with the drug problem. The program providing medical heroin to registered Swiss addicts had been shown to be more effective at reducing crime than policing (Klingemann, 1996; Sabom, 2000).

Social Views, Customs, and Practices

Another interesting factor of the Swiss view of drugs and the drug problem is their treatment of marijuana as a soft drug. In Switzerland, marijuana cultivation goes back hundreds of years. Cannabis was a lucrative cash crop for Swiss farmers until the early 1960s. Nevertheless, when the world panicked over marijuana use by the young, Swiss farmers stopped growing it. Swiss law and treaty of 1961 were, however, never changed to make cultivation illegal in Switzerland.

Few knew and still fewer cared that cannabis was legal in Switzerland until American-Swiss citizen Shirin Patterson uncovered the legal status of cannabis in her research of Swiss laws. Later, in 1993, she formed the Swiss Hemp Trading Company (SWIHTCO) and has since been growing cannabis and informing other Swiss farmers of their right to grow marijuana. Mainly through her efforts, many farmers in Switzerland now belong to the world's largest, most successful agricultural cooperative dedicated to the planting, cultivation, and harvesting of cannabis sativa (Patterson, 1998).

In 1998 SWIHTCO had twelve acres under cultivation, and about fifty additional farmers were growing cannabis in Switzerland. SWIHTCO has been constant in its efforts to promote the production of organic, high-quality cannabis and making it available to anyone and everyone who can benefit from its therapeutic and medicinal use. The Swiss government has not moved with any force to stop the farmers from cultivating marijuana. It is even possible for Switzerland hemp farmers to receive government subsidies for growing marijuana (Patterson, 1998).

Marijuana in Switzerland

Although possessing and using cannabis is not legal per se in Switzerland, there is little or no enforcement of the laws. Although the interest in prosecuting the user varies from Swiss state to Swiss state, penalties on the federal law books range from one day to three months in jail for second-time users who are arrested, and up to three years for users arrested multiple times. These laws were rarely enforced in the late 1990s.

Open marijuana smoking on Swiss streets, in restaurants, or coffee shops is unacceptable. To some degree, this is because the knowledge about the legality of cannabis is not well known. Even so, cannabis flowers are sold over the counter in pharmacies and health food stores throughout Switzerland. No prescription is required; it is found on the shelf with shampoo and vitamin C.

Marijuana stores in Switzerland, with their usual selection of clothing and paraphernalia that reflect a marijuana theme, are growing their own plants and selling buds alongside grow lights. Marijuana plants can also be purchased from farmers in the countryside, and foods available in many open-air markets are made from marijuana buds. "Space cookies" are the best known of these foods (Braben, 2000).

The Range of Hard-Drug Prevention and Treatment Programs

Because the cantons (individual states) control most of the health programs in Switzerland, there is no national system of recording or reporting on drug treatment. However, reports from the cantons give an overview of the drug-treatment services available in Switzerland.

The general trend has been to increase nonresidential services. "Drop-ins" and counseling facilities more than doubled between 1978 and 1988, and they continued to increase into the twenty-first century. A 1993 survey found that twenty-two new facilities had opened between 1989 and 1993. Although not all of the facilities were exclusively for drug users, the increase reflected the rising trend in outpatient treatment (Klingemann, 1996).

The most notable change has been the increase in low-threshold harm-reduction programs, particularly in the later 1980s. As the use of the Platz-spitz (Needle Park) began to grow in 1986, and the incidence of AIDS rose, the medical and social conditions of the drug users deteriorated, and new measures were required. Treatment had long been geared to abstinence; Needle Park was a stark indicator of the failure of that philosophy (Klingemann, 1996). Paradoxically, the high visibility of heroin addicts and the open drug scenes, mainly in Bern and Zurich, resulted in the development of "aid for survival"—low-threshold programs, publicly funded which reached out to heavy heroin users who were living and dying in the city parks but were not ready to seek drug treatment. Specific low-threshold services included shelter, primary medical care, meals, work, needle-exchange facilities, methadone maintenance services for special needs (e.g., institutional services for female prostitutes), and—highly controversial—so-called street rooms or *Gassenzimmer*, injection rooms where intravenous heroin use under hygienic conditions is tolerated and drug dealing is forbidden (Klingemann, 1996).

An example of a low-threshold program drop-in center, which services those who are severely addicted, is a place, without a special room for drug use, which offers free or cheap meals in a cafeteria-type setting. Showers, toilets, and a laundromat are available. Medical care includes the exchange of syringes and a supply of disinfectant cotton swabs. Drugs are not allowed in the center, but there is no demand that the addict abstain or accept treatment to receive the services offered at the drop-in center.

Another example of a low-threshold program is a needle-exchange program. The philosophy of this program is not abstinence, or the reduction of drug use as such; these issues are secondary to the threat of HIV infection and its spread to the greater heterosexual and alcohol-consuming population. This program provides clean syringes and needles, hygienic cotton swabs and vein creams, condoms, tea, and fruit. It also provides primary medical care, hepatitis-B vaccinations, and information on treatment options, as well as instruction in safe sex, hygiene, and health behavior. The needle-exchange rate (new syringes for old) was found to be over 90 percent effective (Klingemann, 1996).

Another valuable low-threshold program is the methadone prescription and maintenance program. In this program, physicians prescribe methadone for identified heroin addicts who cannot quit using heroin. Advocates point out that methadone also promotes social integration and earlier treatment, even without the prospect of abstinence.

The most innovative and controversial low-threshold program is the prescription heroin program. In 1992 the Swiss government passed legislation to make Swiss drug policy more effective. Its intentions were to reduce drug-related harm and the number of users by 20 percent within five years. To accomplish this goal, among other programs, the government authorized a pilot heroin prescription program with a small number of chronic heroin addicts to be scientifically evaluated between 1993 and 1996. The evaluation report, although as controversial as the heroin prescription program, showed a decrease in crime, a decrease in use, and an increase in treatment-seeking among the sample (Farrell and Hall, 1998).

THE FUTURE OF SUBSTANCE ABUSE IN SWITZERLAND

In the near future, the Swiss government could take another advanced step by passing legalization that would issue every Swiss resident over 18 who uses drugs, or who would like to try the different types of drugs available, an electronic credit card to withdraw a specified amount of drugs from a drugstore. The personal dose or amount for each specific drug would be determined for each person in consultation with a doctor or other medical professional. No psychological or medical treatment would be mandated. Both hard drugs and soft drugs would be treated in the same way as alcohol. In other words, the government, if not the medical professionals, will accept the fact that, for some people, addiction is normal, given their physiological circumstances. Although out of line with abstinence and recovery philosophies for adults, in terms of adolescents, people younger than eighteen years of age would be required to see a drug counselor before receiving an electronic drug credit card. The card would be used like an automatic teller machine (ATM) card. In this case, instead of withdrawing cash, the person would withdraw the drug needed from a local drugstore regulated by the state. The appropriate dose for each person would be programmed into the state computer system. The addict or drug-using consumer would run his or her card with its magnetic strip through the machine and the drugstore would supply, for example, a gram of heroin. In 1998 street heroin cost about $32 a gram; prescription heroin sold in a drugstore would cost less than a third of the street price. Users could withdraw drugs daily, or up to one week's supply. Under this program, it is expected that trafficking will disappear because of the legal, cheap, better quality of prescription heroin and other drugs provided by the state. Drug cartels will not have a market and will take their drugs elsewhere to continue earning big drug profits. HIV infection rates among needle users will drop, and the needle-exchange program will provide the addict with the conduit needed to get health services and drug treatment when he or she is ready (Sabom, 2000).

Proposed Solutions and Strategies

Switzerland needs to move forward with decriminalizing soft drugs and providing a separate supply system for soft drugs that does not come into contact with hard drugs; to develop soft-drug policies similar to those used by the Alcohol Board to regulate alcohol; to begin selling soft drugs in state-controlled stores to drive traffickers out of business; to provide heroin and methadone at public-health clinics that provide clean needles, paraphernalia, and a sterile injection room to all addicts who continue to relapse on heroin, thus permitting the monitoring of the health of addicts; and to use identification cards to deter foreign addicts from moving to Switzerland to take advantage of this system.

Other measures include developing prevention programs that are educational in that they show the consequences of misusing a drug, as well as showing ways to use it safely; providing multiple-level treatment upon demand; including outpatient services, drop-in centers, residential long-term treatment, and rehabilitation programs; and continuing to police drug trafficking.

CONCLUSION

Switzerland has moved years closer to decriminalizing drug use and providing services to meet the needs of their drug-addicted citizens. Even so, they could improve their approach by viewing the severely addicted person as a disabled person who can benefit from professional help in learning how to compensate and cope with his or her addiction disability. The disabled addict may need education and added health monitoring while using. If disabled addicts do stop using, their abused bodies will require ongoing medical attention. Even more ominous, probably no one who has ever been addicted to one of the abused drugs (e.g., alcohol, heroin, cocaine, benzodiazepines, barbiturates, tobacco, and even coffee) is ever truly free of the emotional addiction to the drug; he or she is always at risk of going back to the drug. Even so, there are ways for the disabled addict to live a more normal life in a country where substance abuse is handled like a public-health problem (such as auto accidents), and the proposed public policy and interventions are based on a harm-reduction model to drug use and addiction.

REFERENCES

Australia Department of Foreign Affairs and Trade. (2000). *Switzerland*. Barton, Australia: Commonwealth of Australia. Retrieved on November 28, 2000, from the World Wide Web: http://www.dfat.gov.au/geo/switzerland/index. html

Braben, M. (2000). The Swiss cannabis report. Arzo, Switzerland: TAC Ethnobotanical Library. Retrieved on November 28, 2000, from the World Wide Web: http://www.tacethno.com/docs/cannareport.html

Brecher, E.M. (1972). *Licit and illicit drugs*. Boston: Little Brown.

Farrell, M., & Hall, W. (1998). The Swiss heroin trials: Testing alternative approaches. *British Medical Journal, 316*, 639.

Hilowitz, J.E. (Ed.). (1990). *Switzerland in Perspective*. Westport, CT: Greenwood Press.

Huxley, A. (1954). *The doors of perception*. New York: Harper & Brothers.

Institute of Alcohol Studies. (1997). *Switzerland—Country Profile*. London: Author. Retrieved on November 26, 2000, from the World Wide Web: http://www.eurocare.org//profiles/switzerland.htm

Klingemann, H.K.H. (1996). Drug treatment in Switzerland: Harm reduction, decentralization and community response. *Addiction, 91*, 723–736.

Olson, E. (1998, November 28). Crime is key as Swiss vote on legalizing hard drugs. *New York Times*, p. A3.

Osmond, H. (1977). Personal communication at Bryce Hospital. Tuscaloosa, AL.

Patterson, S. (1998, January 2). Visit to the Dream Farm. *Cannabis Culture Magazine*. Retrieved on November 28, 2000, from the World Wide Web: http://www.cannabisculture.com

Sabom, D. (2000). Swiss say yes to doling out heroin. InsightMag.Com (http://www.insightmag.com/archive/200009187.shtml)

Satel, S.L., & Aeschbach, E. (1999). The Swiss heroin trials: Scientifically sound? *Journal of Substance Abuse Treatment, 17*(4), 331–335.

Shields, M. (1998, November 29). *Swiss turn back bid to legalize drugs*. Reuters News Service.

Steinberg, J. (1996). *Why Switzerland?* Cambridge, Eng.: Cambridge University Press.

Strassman, R.J. (1995). Hallucinogenic drugs in psychiatric research and treatment: Perspective and prospects. *Journal of Nervous and Mental Disease, 183*(3), 127–138.

Swiss Alcohol Board. (2000). *Alcohol consumption—Facts and effects*. Berne: Swiss Alcohol Board. Retrieved on November 30, 2000, from the World Wide Web: http://www.eav.admin.ch/e/f_konsu.htm.

Swiss Federal Office of Public Health. (1999). *Facts and figures on the drug problem*. Berne: Swiss Federal Office of Public Health. http://www.admin.ch/bag/sucth/epi/e/facts-e.htm.

13

UNITED STATES

Douglas Rugh

INTRODUCTION

Understanding the scope of drug use and addiction in the world includes knowing the prevalence among various populations and researching the many health and social consequences. The United States is both the largest producer of drug research in the world and the world's only "drug-control superpower." The simultaneous leadership in social science and world agenda setting is not the result of a symbiotic relationship between American research and policy making. This chapter summarizes the research perspective of the United States of America and outlines the current policies associated with controlling the country's drug problem.

General Characteristics of Alcohol and Drug Addiction

Dramatic scientific advances primarily in the United States over the past two decades have revolutionized our understanding of drug use and addiction. Foremost among these advances is a clear understanding that drug use is a preventable behavior and that drug addiction is a treatable disease of the brain. This approach runs counter to the broadly held view in the United States that addicts are so incapacitated by drugs that they are unable to modify any of their behaviors. Research has shown that drug use as a health issue is a double-edged sword. It affects both the health of the individual and the health of society. For individuals, the use of drugs has well-known and severe negative consequences for both mental and physical health. For the U.S. public, drug use and addiction have tremendous negative implications for the health of the individual and society. In the United States, drug use is a major factor in violent crimes, and it is a vector for the transmission of serious infectious diseases, particularly AIDS, hepatitis, and tuberculosis. Drug use destroys family relationships. It leads to domestic violence, child neglect, and child abuse. Drugs interfere with education and increase the chances of income loss.

An accurate understanding of the nature of drug use and addiction in the United States and other countries should also include an understanding of the role the criminal justice system can play in reducing addiction. For example, if we know that criminals are drug addicted, it is no longer reasonable simply to incarcerate them. If they have a brain disease (as proposed by many U.S. scientists), imprisoning them without treatment is futile. If they are left untreated, their chances of returning to a life of crime and drug use are high. However, studies have shown that when addicted criminals are treated, both types of recidivism can be reduced dramatically.

Understanding addiction as a brain disease also affects how society approaches and deals with addicted individuals. Even if drug use started as voluntary behavior, an addict's brain is different from a nonaddict's brain. The addicted individual is in a different or diseased brain state. As recently as the beginning of the twentieth century, individuals with schizophrenia were put in prison-like asylums; we know now that they require medical treatment. Medication helps to alleviate symptoms associated with the altered brain function, and the therapeutic environment helps the concomitant behavioral and social functioning components of this illness.

Understanding addiction as a brain disease explains in part the failure of historic strategies that have focused on the criminal justice aspects of drug use and addiction. If the brain is at the core of the problem, attending to and treating the brain must be the core solution. At the beginning of the twenty-first century, ever-changing drug-use patterns, the continuing transmission of HIV infection among drug users, and the need to develop effective treatment and preventive interventions underscore the importance of research in finding new and better ways to alleviate the pain and devastation of addiction. Never before has there existed a greater need to increase our knowledge about drug use.

Treating Addiction

Because addiction is such a complex and pervasive health issue, we must include in our overall strategies a committed public health approach that includes extensive education and prevention efforts, treatment, and research. Drug addiction, like heart disease, can be a serious, life-threatening disease. However, it is treatable by a combination of medications and behavioral therapies. One goal of drug-addiction treatment in the United States is no different from the goal of treating heart disease: to prolong and improve the patient's quality of life. Over the years, U.S. researchers have amassed an impressive amount of scientific knowledge about the treatment of drug use and addiction. This research has clearly shown that drug-abuse treatment can reduce drug use, drug-related criminal behavior, and therefore the health and social costs of drug use and addiction. Modern approaches to treating addiction have benefited from two types of studies. Longitudinal studies of large populations have helped us identify behavioral and social antecedents to drug use that can be targets for therapeutic intervention. At the same time, neurobiological studies have elucidated the molecular underpinnings of addictive behavior and, in doing so, have identified numerous targets for drug development efforts. The result of this concerted effort is a host of new therapies, both behavioral and pharmacological, which can effectively treat many aspects of drug use and addiction.

Individual Traits

Many individual-level factors, which place youth at risk for or protect them from using illicit drugs, have been identified. Recent research indicates that personality and behavioral traits and styles, evident in early childhood, may have implications for later substance-use behaviors. One such trait is aggressiveness (Dodge, Lochman, Harnish, et al., 1997).

Gender may also play a role in substance abuse. In general, females are less likely to use illicit substances than males. However, some subgroups of females may be at heightened risk. For example, Latino girls in the United States are at greater risk of receiving drug offers than females from other ethnic groups (Hecht, Trost, Bator, et al., 1997).

A number of indicators have been identified as strong predictors of later abuse. One indicator is a young age at drug initiation. A second indicator is a strong association between a young person's perception of low levels of competency in school and starting to use tobacco and alcohol in elementary school. It also appears that the teacher's perception of the student's competency is associated with abusive behaviors (Jackson, 1997). Over time, these perceptions begin to act as self-fulfilling prophecies. High school students in the United States, who were more susceptible to social influences and displayed lower levels of competency, were more likely to exhibit increased drinking behavior (Scheier, Botvin, and Baker, 1997). Besides the important role of perception, these data demonstrate a stable set of individual factors which relate to the initiation and progression of substance use over the course of development.

By late adolescence, increased drug use contributes to impaired social, emotional, and psychological development. As a further complication, memory associations of drug cues and drug use influence future decisions to use drugs (Stacy, Galaif, Sussman, et al., 1996). One group of scientists speculates that cognitive deficits may actually precede and predispose some individuals to drug-use initiation. Thus, weaknesses in cognitive skills and learning disabilities may be undetected risk factors that underlie other identified risk factors, such as low self-esteem and academic failure.

Research is beginning to show that the developmental stages of drug involvement are not identical for males and females. In the progression from legal drug use to illicit drug use, for example, cigarettes have a relatively larger role for females than for males, and alcohol has a relatively larger role for males than for females. With regard to initiation into illicit drugs, data suggest that women are more likely to begin or maintain cocaine use as a way to develop intimate relationships. Men are more likely to use the drugs with male friends and become involved with drug trafficking. The onset of drug abuse occurs later for females, and the paths are more complex than for males. For females, there is typically a pattern of breakdown of individual, familial, and environmental protective factors and an increase in childhood fears, anxieties, phobias, and failed relationships.

Childhood sexual abuse has been associated with drug use in females in several studies. Some studies indicate that as many as 70 percent of women report histories of physical and sexual abuse, with victimization beginning before eleven years of age and occurring repeatedly. A study of drug use among young women who became pregnant before reaching eighteen years of age reported that 32 percent had a history of early forced sexual intercourse (rape or incest) [Dembo, et al., 1987]. These adolescents, compared with nonvictims, used more crack, cocaine, and other drugs (except marijuana); had lower self-esteem; and engaged in a higher number of delinquent activities (Jackson, 1997). Furthermore, female drug users may have greater vulnerability to victimization than males. For example, in a recent study of homicide in New York City, 59 percent of white women and 72 percent of African-American women had been using cocaine before death compared with 38 percent of white men and 44 percent of African-American men. Thus, although more males than females use cocaine in the United States, its use is a far greater risk factor for the victimization of women than men (Gondolf, 1995). Therefore, it is critical that the factors involved in the relationship between drug use and dependence among females and physical and sexual victimization (including partner violence) be identified and understood.

The rate of co-occurring substance-use disorders and other psychiatric disorders is relatively high for U.S. females. Data from a study on female crime victims, for example, indicate that those suffering from posttraumatic stress disorder (PTSD) were seventeen times more likely to have major drug-use problems than nonvictims (Fullilove, et al., 1993). In addition, individuals with a trauma history and PTSD use drugs more frequently than do their non-PTSD counterparts. This fact has led researchers to speculate that the co-occurrence of substance use and PTSD may predict a more severe course than would ordinarily be present with either disorder alone. For females, a high correlation appears to exist between eating disorders and substance use. For example, as many as 55 percent of bulimic patients are reported to have drug- and alcohol-abuse problems. Conversely, as many as 40 percent of females with drug-use or alcohol problems have been reported to have eating disorder syndromes, usually involving binge eating (Brooner, King, Kidorf, et al., 1997). In one recent U.S. study, psychiatric and substance use co-morbidity was assessed in opiate abusers seeking methadone maintenance. Rates of co-occurring mental disorders and personality traits were compared by gender, and the results showed that women were more likely than men to have a mood disorder and were seven times more likely than men to have a borderline personality disorder. Although all patients had at least one substance-use diagnosis beyond opiate dependence, most often cocaine dependence, women were less likely than men to have a lifetime marijuana, alcohol, or hallucinogen disorder or current marijuana or alcohol dependence (Brooner, King, Kidorf, et al., 1997).

Family Traits

Parenting practices are central to children's being put at risk for drug use. To understand developmental patterns leading to adolescent drug use, scientists have focused extensively on the role of parenting in establishing, maintaining, or exacerbating risk in children and adolescents. Early onset is not random. It is often a predictable and identifiable progression that begins in early childhood. A child's development involves the interaction of the child's characteristics with the context of the family. It is not so much who the parents are but what skills they bring to the socialization of the child that is the most important factor (Dishion, Kavanagh, and Kiesner, 1998). A number of studies have shown that poor parental monitoring and parent-child conflict predict the initial use and trajectory of alcohol, tobacco, and marijuana use (Duncan, Duncan, Biglan, et al., 1998). In fact, parental monitoring is linked both directly and indirectly to the early onset of drug use: directly, through the lack of actual supervision, and indirectly, through the additional time spent with peers. In the United States, children who are not monitored tend to loiter in areas where drug use and other delinquent activities might occur (Dishion, Kavanagh, and Kiesner, 1998). Parenting practices can serve a protective role in the face of adverse environments.

The social model of childhood development hypothesizes that strong emotional bonds to adults and to institutions associated with antisocial behavior contribute to the development of antisocial behavior. Consistent with this perspective, research has indicated that children who bond strongly to substance-using parents are at risk of developing alcohol or drug problems themselves (Colder, Lochman, and Wells, 1997). This information demonstrates the importance of bonding for the prediction of problematic behaviors. Bonding has also been established as a protective factor against future drug or alcohol use. For instance, strong bonds with a drug-free adult, educational goals, or a sports club can mitigate the effects of poverty, destructive peer pressure, or genetics.

Scientists have found that between 25 and 50 percent of men who act violently within the home have substance-abuse problems (Gondolf, 1995). A recent survey of public child welfare agencies, conducted by the National Committee to Prevent Child Abuse, found that as many as eighty percent of child abuse cases are associated with the use of alcohol and drugs (McCurdy and Daro, 1994). The link between child abuse and other forms of domestic violence in the United States is well established. Research also indicates that women who abuse alcohol or drugs are more likely to become victims of family violence (Miller, Downs, and Gondoli, 1989). Survivors are more likely to become dependent on tranquilizers, sedatives, stimulants, and painkillers. They also are more likely to abuse alcohol (Stark and Flitcraft, 1988).

The connection between substance abuse and family violence also includes

- About 40 percent of children from violent homes believe that their fathers had a drinking problem and that they were more abusive when drinking (Roy, 1988).
- Childhood physical abuse is associated with later substance abuse by youth (Dembo, Dertke, LaVoie, et al., 1987).
- Alcoholic women are more likely to report a history of childhood physical and emotional abuse than are nonalcoholic women (Hein and Scheier, 1996).
- Women in recovery are likely to have a history of violent trauma and are at high risk of being diagnosed with PTSD (Fullilove, Fullilove, Smith, et al., 1993).

Impact on Pregnancy

One aspect of drug use by women that is of particular concern is the use of drugs during pregnancy. Research indicates that pregnant drug users are at increased risk for miscarriage, tubal pregnancy, stillbirth, low weight gain, anemia, hypertension, and other medical problems. In addition, newborns may have lower birth weight and a smaller head size than babies born to non–drug using mothers. Among the total cases of pediatric AIDS in the United States, 54% are related to either maternal injection drug use or maternal sex with an injecting drug user (Hershow, Riester, Lew, et al., 1997).

Profile of the United States

At the turn of the twenty-first century, the United States of America is one of the most powerful nations on earth. It has great wealth in natural resources, and many of its citizens have accumulated vast personal fortunes. Even so, this enormous wealth has not translated into benefits for many of its citizens who are poor and disadvantaged. Although leading other nations in the production of manufactured goods, technology, higher education, and military hardware, the United States usually lags behind other industrial nations in providing for the social needs of its citizens, especially its poor.

The population in the United States in 1998 was 270,311,758 with a labor force of 134,125,342. People of European descent constitute about 84 percent of the population; African descent, 13 percent; Asians and Pacific Islanders, 3 percent; and Native Americans, about 1 percent. Hispanics, who may also be counted among other groups, make up about 9 percent (*Encarta Desk Encyclopedia*, 1998).

Approximately 75 percent of the people live in urban areas. The capital is Washington, D.C. The government, a federal republic with a strong democratic tradition was founded in 1776 when, through revolution, it broke away from England and became an independent country. (*Encarta Desk Encyclopedia*, 1998).

The gross domestic product (GDP) in 1995 was 8.5 trillion dollars, or $31,500 per person. In 1997 the military consumed 3.4 percent of the national GDP, and, in the same year, the active troop strength was 1.55 million (*Encarta Desk Encyclopedia*, 1998).

There are 146 million passenger cars and another 59 million commercial vehicles in use in the United States, or 1 vehicle for every 1.3 persons in the United States. There are 834 airports with scheduled flights in the United State. There is 1 television set per 1.2 persons and 2 radios for each person; there is also 1 telephone per 1.7 people in the United States (*Encarta Desk Encyclopedia*, 1998).

The life expectancy at birth in the United States in 1996 was seventy-three years of age for males and seventy-nine years of age for females. There were fifteen births per 1,000 people and nine deaths per 1,000 people. There is one hospital bed for every 223 people and one physician for every 391 persons. Infant mortality is seven per 1,000 live births, but it is much higher for some minority groups and the poor (*Encarta Desk Encyclopedia*, 1998).

In the United States, 86.5 percent of the population are Christian (Baptist, Episcopalian, Lutheran, Methodist, Roman Catholic, and other Christian religious groups). Jewish religious groups make up 1.8 percent; Muslims 0.5 percent; and Buddhist and Hindu, less than 0.5 percent (*Encarta Desk Encyclopedia*, 1998).

Elementary and secondary education is free and compulsory. The duration of compulsory education is ten years between the ages of seven and sixteen. Approximately 96 percent of people in the United States are officially literate (*Encarta Desk Encyclopedia*, 1998).

VIGNETTE

Judy, a white high school graduate in her late twenties, is trying to recover from severe cocaine addiction. She is a survivor of rape and violence. Her story is typical of the many problems and circumstances faced by women who enter the substance abuse treatment systems.

Judy's uncle molested her from the age of three until she was ten. The molestation included vaginal penetration. Like many other victims of sexual abuse, Judy was threatened by her abuser, and she never disclosed the abuse. On one occasion, her mother asked her whether her uncle had ever touched her, and she replied, "No, he does nice things for me."

At age fifteen, she became sexually active with her twenty-three-year-old boyfriend, Alex. Together they began using marijuana. When she was eighteen, she started using cocaine with Alex, who was now occasionally slapping her and forcing her to have sex.

She discovered she was pregnant. She decided to have the baby but received only sporadic prenatal care. During her pregnancy, both Judy and Alex used cocaine and marijuana and drank alcohol. The infant, a girl named Candace, was born at full term but was small for her gestational age. Alex left Judy soon thereafter, and she and Candace moved in with a new boyfriend, Billy. He used drugs and was both extremely possessive and violent. He intimidated Judy and sometimes threatened to kill her, Candace, and himself.

When Candace was three, Judy, then twenty-one, became pregnant again. Billy did not welcome the pregnancy and began hitting her in the abdomen and breasts when he was angry. Judy received no prenatal care during her second pregnancy and delivered a preterm baby whom she named Patricia.

By the time Patricia was born, Judy's drug use had escalated to include crack and increasing amounts of alcohol. Despite her mounting problems, Judy recognized that her new baby was a poor feeder. Judy was frightened enough to keep a six-week post-delivery pediatric visit during which Patricia was diagnosed as "failing to thrive." At the same visit, three-year-old Candace was weighed and found to be only in the tenth percentile of weight for her age.

Two weeks later, Judy and Billy were arrested on drug charges—Judy for possession and Billy for dealing. She received probation, and she and her children moved in with her mother, Vivian. Billy was incarcerated, and Judy was required by the court to participate in substance-abuse treatment.

In a group therapy session in her substance-abuse treatment program, Judy acknowledged her history of family violence, childhood sexual abuse, and battering. Her case manager in this program wanted her to join another group of childhood incest survivors, but Judy felt ashamed and did not want to discuss the incest further. She began attending treatment sessions sporadically and, after two months, dropped out. In the meantime, tension developed between Judy and Vivian. Judy felt that her mother cared more for her granddaughters than she had about Judy when she was a child. Now that Judy had acknowledged her history of sexual abuse, she found herself blaming her mother for "allowing" it to happen. She also was jealous because she felt that Vivian was a better mother to Patricia and Candace than she was. After a series of violent fights with her mother, Judy moved out and got a minimum-wage job, leaving her children with Vivian.

Around this time, Judy met Cody, a drug dealer. Cody moved in with her, but frequent arguing and mutual battering characterized their relationship. Judy's work habits became erratic; she often had bruises and sprains that she refused to discuss when her concerned coworkers questioned her about them. Although she saw her children infrequently, she called late at night when she was high and criticized Vivian for keeping her children from her.

For a brief time, Judy's life appeared to stabilize. Although she had not finished her substance-abuse treatment program, she and Cody were both working, and she continued to receive negative screens for drugs (although she was still using occasionally). At the next child protective services hearing, the children were returned to Judy's custody with the stipulation that she participate in parenting classes as well as continue in treatment.

As soon as her two children moved in with her and Cody, the situation began to deteriorate. Cody could not tolerate the children, and his episodes of violent behavior increased. He put his fist through the wall and kicked the door down. He became increasingly angry at Judy's frequent absences because of "all this kid stuff" (parenting classes and Candace's preschool program). He began to "spank" the children or grab them roughly by their arms when he wanted their attention. They showed up at their respective day care and preschool programs with bruises, which were attributed to "accidents." No one at the day care or preschool programs was aware of Judy's history or her disclosures of childhood abuse and battering in the treatment program.

Cody's violence continued to escalate and, increasingly, was directed at the children. Although Judy was concerned about his hitting and yelling at the children, she did not know what to do about it. She was feeling overwhelmed by her job, the parenting classes, her meetings with social services workers and her probation officer, and her child care responsibilities. In time, however, she began intervening when Cody yelled at or hit the children, deliberately provoking him in order to divert his attention away from the children and onto herself. The neighbors called 911 frequently, but the police never found any substantial evidence of violence.

A year passed with no improvement. The children continued to attend school, but Judy appeared only sporadically at her parenting classes and the preschool program. She was now beginning to suspect that Cody was sexually abusing five-year-old Candace. Judy had begun to notice the same kinds of behavior in her daughter that she remembered in herself when she was sexually abused at that age. One day she asked Candace whether Cody had ever touched her in certain ways. Candace replied, "No, he is always nice to me." Judy remembered using almost identical words to her own mother years before and was certain that her daughter was being victimized in the same way. All the rage from her own abuse by her uncle erupted. She confronted Cody and a battle developed, which Candace witnessed. Later this episode became a major treatment issue for the child, who believed that the violence in her household was her fault.

Without a safe haven for Judy, her drug use will continue and her life will continue to be in jeopardy. At this point, residential treatment is the only option that will save the lives of Cody, Judy, and the children. Cody's criminal charges resulted in his being sentenced to jail and, after release, residential treatment.

OVERVIEW OF PROBLEM IN THE UNITED STATES AND BASIC DEMOGRAPHICS

Drug crimes receive some of the severest criminal sanctions in the U.S. legal system. Based on federal surveys and by definition of the current laws, more than 50 percent of all high school seniors are drug criminals who should be imprisoned. Is this a realistic or an appropriate approach to controlling juvenile drug use?

Programming and Special Populations

Preventive interventions in the United States appear to be most effective when they consider characteristics, risk, and protective factors associated with the target group. Thus, efforts are being made to understand what risk and protective factors may be salient for specific racial and ethnic groups and subgroups. For example, among middle school children, Latino males and females were more likely to experience drug offers than other students. However, there were no differences in the type or setting of drug offers. For all groups, offers were simple, rather than complex and pressure filled, and could be resisted with simple refusals. Drugs tended to be offered to all groups most frequently at home and in public settings rather than at school or at parties. In another sample of 448 Latino young adolescents, increased interaction with non-Latino peers was positively related to attitudes and perceived peer norms against substance use (Hecht, Trost, Bator, et al., 1997).

The patient-centered self-help fellowship of men and women called Alcoholics Anonymous allows its members to share their common experience and thus to help each other. It is a voluntary fellowship of alcoholic persons who seek to get sober and remain sober through self-help and the support of recovered alcoholics. AA began in May 1935 when two men met to overcome their drinking problems: a New York stockbroker, "Bill W." (William Griffith Wilson [1895–1971]), and a surgeon from Akron, Ohio, "Dr. Bob S." (Robert Holbrook Smith [1879–1950]). The members strive to follow a series of Twelve Steps. The central points rely on God or a higher power. Although general conventions meet periodically and Alcoholics Anonymous World Services, Inc., is headquartered in New York City, all AA groups are essentially local and autonomous. To counteract self-indulgence and promote the group's welfare, members identify themselves only by first name and surname initial. Much of the program has a social and spiritual, but nonsectarian, basis.

By the late twentieth century, Alcoholics Anonymous had approximately 2 million members in about 90,000 groups in 122 countries and territories (most of them in the United States and Canada). The fellowship is organized in local groups of indeterminate size, has no dues, and accepts contributions for its expenses only from those attending meetings, where members narrate the stories of their alcoholic careers and their recovery in AA.

AA apparently meets the needs of its members by enabling them to associate with people who understand them, to accept the disease concept of alcoholism, to admit their powerlessness over alcohol and their need for help, to depend without shame or stigma on others, and to involve themselves in activities within the group and in helping other alcoholics. These goals attempt to provide adequate substitutes for the alcohol-dependent way of life. AA is thought by many to be the single most successful method yet devised for coping with alcoholism. It has spawned some allied but independent organizations: Al-Anon, for spouses and other close relatives and friends of alcoholics; Narcotics Anonymous (NA), for those addicted to any narcotics; and Alateen, for adolescent children of alcoholics. Professionals in the field tend to think of AA as an inexpensive form of group therapy and a useful ally, but recognize, as do the more sophisticated members, that it is not a panacea and it is not suitable for all types of alcoholics. Most experienced therapists agree, however, that any form of treatment is likely to show a higher rate of success if the patient can be persuaded simultaneously to join Alcoholics Anonymous.

U.S. Demographics and Statistics

This section presents some of the most recent findings from three major sources of epidemiological data on drug use. It also provides a perspective on patterns and trends in drug use. The Monitoring the Future (MTF) Study and the Community Epidemiology Work Group (CEWG) Study are sponsored by the National Institute on Drug Abuse (NIDA). The National Household Survey on Drug Abuse (NHSDA) is administered by the Substance Abuse and Mental Health Services Administration (SAMHSA), U.S. Department of Health and Human Services.

The 1997 NHSDA found that an estimated 13.9 million Americans twelve years and older had used an illicit drug in the month before the interview. Many more people try drugs than go on to become regular users. Although NHSDA survey results show that nearly 36 percent of all Americans older than age eleven have tried any illicit drug during their lifetimes, only 11 percent have used any illicit drug during the past year, and only 6 percent have used any illicit drug during the past month. This same finding holds true for specific illicit drugs. In their lifetimes, 33 percent of Americans age twelve or older have smoked marijuana at least once, but only 5.1 percent used marijuana during the past month. Although the overall numbers are higher, the same trend holds true for cigarette use. Nearly 71 percent of Americans report that they had smoked a cigarette at some time in their lives, but only 30 percent reported having smoked a cigarette during the past month. These findings show the importance of identifying both the factors that place people at risk for drug use and the protective factors that keep many people from becoming regular users (SAMHSA, 1998).

Rates of illicit drug use vary by ethnicity and gender. Most current illicit drug users are white non-Hispanics, a group that accounts for 74 percent of all users. However, the rate of current illicit drug use for blacks (7.5 percent of the black population) remains somewhat higher than for whites (6.4 percent of the white non-Hispanic population) and Hispanics (5.9 percent of the Hispanic population). However, among youth the rates of use are about the same for all three major U.S. ethnic groups. As has been true for some time now, in 1997, men continued to have a higher rate of current illicit drug use than women (8.5 percent of men versus 4.5 percent of women). However, among twelve- to seventeen-year-old drug users, there was little difference in the rate of drug use between adolescent males and females (9.2 percent for males versus 8.9 percent for females). Rates of illicit drug use in 1997 also show substantial variation by age and educational status. Among youths ages twelve and thirteen, 3.8 percent were current illicit drug users. The highest rates were found among young people ages sixteen and seventeen (19.2 percent) and ages eighteen to twenty (17.3 percent). Rates of use were lower in each successive age group, with only about 1 percent of people age 50 and older reporting current illicit use. Among young adults ages eighteen to thirty-four, those who had not completed high school had the highest rate of current use (14.1 percent); college graduates had the lowest rate of use (5.9 percent). This is despite the fact that young adults at different educational levels are equally likely to have tried illicit drugs in their lifetimes. Illicit drug use also varies by geographic location. In 1997 the current illicit drug use rate was 8.1 percent in the West, 7.3 percent in the North Central, 5.8 percent in the South, and 4.7

percent in the Northeast. Rates were higher in metropolitan areas than in nonmetropolitan areas (SAMHSA, 1998).

HISTORY OF ALCOHOL AND DRUG ABUSE IN THE UNITED STATES

Alcohol, the most conspicuous drug of concern in the United States, seemingly was at the root of such other social problems as unemployment, crime, and violence. "Ministers shall not give themselves to excess in drinkinge, or riott, or spending their tyme idellye day or night," ruled the Virginia Colonial Assembly in 1629 (Cherrington, 1920, p. 16). Massachusetts ordered that no person shall remain in any tavern "longer than necessary occasions" in 1637, while Plymouth Colony in 1633 prohibited the sale of spirits "more than 2 pence worth to anyone but strangers just arrived" (Cherrington, 1920, p. 18). This sampling of the earliest colonial laws is representative of the attempt, continued since those times, to control excessive consumption. Excessive drinking, it was considered, produced behavior unseemly in some, such as ministers, and dangerous in others, such as Indians.

The regulation of liquor consumption was a matter of considerable concern in certain colonies. Thus, for a time, Massachusetts went so far as to prohibit the drinking of toasts in 1638 (Lee, 1963). The law was soon abandoned because of the difficulties associated with enforcing a complete ban. It rapidly became clear that liquor laws could do more than control consumption: they could provide a source of revenue. By the turn of the eighteenth century, the regulatory impulse was concentrated on fines, excise taxes, and license fees.

The anger of the movement was epitomized by the travels of Father Theobald Matthew of Ireland who toured the United States from 1849 to 1851, administering the pledge of total abstinence to some 600,000 persons in twenty-five states. A White House dinner and a Senate reception stamped official approval upon his sojourns (Furnas, 1965). Temperance thus entered a new phase. It was in this atmosphere that the first prohibition experiments were undertaken on a statewide basis.

Despite the lack of support from the general population and the disagreements among the state legislatures, by 1902, the temperance campaign had permeated the public school systems. Every state but Arizona had introduced compulsory temperance education. Their texts teemed with both facts and misinformation such as, "Alcohol sometimes causes the coats of the blood vessels to grow thin. They are then liable at any time to cause death by bursting" (Sinclair, 1962, p. 43).

As scientists began accumulating evidence of the effect of quantities of alcohol on the nervous system and general physical condition, the myth that alcohol consumption improved muscular power was disproved. The relationship between mental psychoses and alcohol was documented, and thus the condemnation of alcohol as a poison had scientific support. Finally, in 1915, whiskey and brandy were discreetly removed from the list of authoritative medicinal drugs contained in the United States Pharmacopoeia (Timberlake, 1963).

The early experience of the Prohibition era gave the government a taste of what was to come. In the three months before the Eighteenth Amendment became effective, liquor worth half a million dollars was stolen from government warehouses. By midsummer of 1920, federal courts in Chicago were overwhelmed with some 600 pending liquor violation trials (Sinclair, 1962). Within three years, thirty prohibition agents were killed in service.

Other statistics demonstrated the increasing volume of the bootleg trade. In 1921, 95,933 illicit distilleries, stills, still works, and fermentors were seized. In 1925, the total jumped to 172,537 and went up to 282,122 in 1930. In connection with these seizures, 34,175 persons were arrested in 1921; by 1925, the number had risen to 62,747; in 1928, a high of 75,307. Concurrently, convictions for liquor offenses in federal courts rose from 35,000 in 1923 to 61,383 in 1932 (Internal Revenue Service, 1921, p. 95; 1966, p. 6; 1970, p. 73).

This trend is similar to the criminalization trend that we see today. The law could not stop the high demand for alcoholic products. When legal enterprises could no longer supply the demand, an illicit network developed, from the point of manufacture to consumption (Lee, 1963).

THE SUBSTANCE ABUSE PROBLEM IN THE UNITED STATES TODAY

Political and Public Policies and Views

Some scholars maintain that U.S. drug policy is *pharmaco-centric*, meaning that it wrongly assumes that the problem lies with the substances, not the people and their social, cultural, ideological, and economic environments. Thus, many social scientists say that policy has been geared toward suppressing the symptoms of deeper social problems in U.S. society rather than attacking the root causes, which explains the failure of government action. In their view, drugs have been singled out as a convenient scapegoat on which to blame and explain away some of the more disturbing problems experienced by American society. But yet another school of research suggests that this assertion is flawed because drug-control policy is not aimed at controlling drugs but rather the "dangerous classes" with which American mainstream society has historically associated them. Drugs have given rise to a culture of terror that can be viewed as an internalized and self-imposed mechanism of control.

The United States enforces an extreme form of total drug prohibition. Although there is de facto decriminalization of marijuana possession in some states and increasing support for medical marijuana use in other states, for the most part, policies in the United States are uniformly prohibitionist in nature. There are few needle-exchange programs. Some states still have laws against the selling of needles without a prescription. There is widespread drug testing, both in the workplace and in schools. Very harsh penalties for all drug offenses apply, with sentencing according to strict mandatory minimum guidelines. The results of this system include continuing very high levels of drug use (some of the highest in the world); escalation of costs to society; an extremely high prevalence of HIV and other diseases, especially among drug users (some of the highest rates in the Western world); and rapid prison expansion. The impact of the prohibition of illegal drugs in the United States in the late twentieth century on U.S. society is similar to the impact of the U.S. prohibition of alcohol in the early part of the twentieth century. For example, despite a fivefold increase in federal expenditures for drug-supply reduction efforts since 1996, cocaine is cheaper today than it was a decade ago, and heroin purity exceeds 60 percent compared to 30 percent in 1990 (Riley, 1998).

In October, Amnesty International released a strongly worded report on the human rights record of the United States. Amnesty International accuses the United States of using double standards and creating a climate "in which human rights violations thrive." The report attacks the United States for what it calls "a persistent and widespread pattern of human rights violations." U.S. federal and state authorities, police, immigration, and prison officers are all criticized in the report, which documents numerous cases of generalized gratuitous violence, sexual abuse, and cruelty. Many of the violations identified by Amnesty International are related to the enforcement of drug laws. More than 50 percent of the incarcerations in the United States are drug related. Conditions in American prisons come in for particular criticism in the Amnesty report. The number of people in U.S. jails has tripled since 1980 to more than 2 million in 2000. Chains and leg-irons are commonly used as restraints despite being prohibited by international law. They also point out that up to one-third of all young black men are in jail or on parole or probation. "We felt it was ironic that the most powerful country in the world uses international human rights laws to criticize others but does not apply the same standards at home" (Riley, 1998, p. 49).

Despite America's drug war, worldwide opium and cocaine production has doubled in the last ten years. The number of countries producing drugs has also doubled. Pressure to end production in one country only increases production in another. Since a single 35-square kilometer plot is enough to grow all the opium consumed in the United States, the likelihood that the United States will stop production is very small indeed. Borders are not easily sealed when it is estimated that one loaded DC3 plane can carry a year's supply of heroin to the United States and twelve trailer trucks can carry enough cocaine across the border to meet the needs of the United States for a year (Riley, 1998).

In 1980, the federal budget for drug control was approximately $1 billion, and state and local budgets were two or three times that. By 1997 the federal drug-control budget had reached $16 billion, two-thirds of it for law enforcement agencies; state and local funding had also increased to at least that level. "These are the results of a drug policy over reliant on criminal justice 'solutions', ideologically wedded to abstinence-only treatment, and insulated from a cost-benefit analysis" (Riley, 1998, p. 49).

Government Recognition and Strategies of Prevention

The National Institute of Drug Addiction (NIDA), which supports more than 85 percent of the world's research on drug use and addiction, continues to identify new technologies and avenues for developing prevention and treatment of drug addiction. These approaches significantly reduce the devastating health and societal effects of drug use and addiction.

NIDA's comprehensive, multidisciplinary prevention research program examines multiple factors which contribute to drug abuse and how these factors interact. The institute has also taken a strong role in synthesizing and disseminating the findings. Recently, the institute released a set of Prevention Principles, which enumerate what has been learned through twenty years of research on what works in keeping children and adolescents from using illicit drugs. The principles that follow can be found in NIDA's *Preventing Drug Use among Children and Adolescents* research-based guide (Sloboda and David, 2000):

1. Prevention programs should be designed to enhance "protective factors" and to move toward reversing or reducing known "risk factors."

2. Prevention programs should target all forms of drug use, including the use of tobacco, alcohol, marijuana, and inhalants.

3. Prevention programs should include skills to resist drugs when offered, strengthen personal commitments against drug use, and increase social competency (e.g., in communications, peer relationships, self-efficacy, and assertiveness) in conjunction with reinforcement of attitudes against drug use.

4. Prevention programs for adolescents should include interactive methods, such as peer discussion groups, rather than didactic teaching techniques alone.

5. Prevention programs should include a parent's or caregiver's component that reinforces what the children are learning, such as facts about drugs and their harmful effects. Moreover, the intervention should promote opportunities for family discussions about use of legal and illegal substances and family policies about their use.

6. Prevention programs should be long term and should continue over the school career, with repeated interventions to reinforce the original prevention goals. For example, school-based efforts directed at elementary school and middle school students should include booster sessions to help with critical transitions from middle school to high school.

7. Family-focused prevention efforts have a greater impact than strategies that focus on parents only or children only.

8. Community programs that include media campaigns and policy changes, such as new regulations that restrict access to alcohol, tobacco, or other drugs, are more effective when they are accompanied by school and by family interventions.

9. Community programs need to strengthen norms against drug use in all drug use prevention settings, including the family, school, and community.

10. Schools offer opportunities to reach all populations and also serve as important settings for specific subpopulations at risk for drug use, such as children with behavior problems or learning disabilities and those who are potential dropouts.

11. Prevention programming should be adapted to address the specific nature of the drug use problem in the local community.

12. The higher the level of risk for the target population, the more intensive the prevention effort must be, and the earlier it must begin.

13. Prevention programs should be age-specific, developmentally appropriate, and culturally sensitive.

14. Effective prevention programs are cost-effective.

Historically U.S. policy has been largely immune from the influence of research, even government-funded research, while a vast proportion of American social science research on drugs has been focused primarily on policy, which has been viewed as a crucial element of America's drug problem. While the government has not been able to achieve its official objective of reducing drug abuse, current U.S. drug policy has resulted in the imprisonment of a large proportion of the American population, mostly poor members of ethnic and racial minorities. Researchers have found that the causal relationship between drugs and crime, which serves as the basis and rationale for present policies, has been vastly exaggerated. In addition, the stringent law-and-order approach adopted by the various levels of U.S. government has been found to be too costly, while its enforcement has led to what appears to be widespread human rights abuse and charges of racial and ethnic prejudice that historians say have been a permanent feature of American drug control since its origins in the late nineteenth century.

Social Views, Customs, and Practices

Women have a difficult time getting help for alcohol or drug addiction. Women who abuse drugs face a variety of barriers, including barriers to treatment entry, treatment engagement, and long-term recovery. Barriers to entry include a lack of economic resources, referral networks, women-oriented services, and conflicting child-related responsibilities. Because women have many specific needs, a number of components of treatment have been found to be important in attracting and retaining women in treatment. These components include the availability of female-sensitive services; nonpunitive, noncoercive treatment which incorporates supportive behavioral change approaches; and treatment for a wide range of medical problems, mental disorders, and psychosocial problems.

One research study showed that the treatment of drug-dependent women was more likely to be successful if treatment was provided in a mutually supportive therapeutic environment and addressed the following issues: psychopathology, such as depression; a woman's role as mother; interpersonal relationships; and the need for parenting education. Another study found that cocaine-using women whose children were living with them during residential treatment remained in the programs significantly longer than women whose children were not living with them at the facility. In this study, approximately 77 percent of the women with their children living in the treatment facility were still in the program at three months, compared with 45 percent of the group that did not have their children with them. At six months, the corresponding figures were 65 percent compared with 18 percent. The clear implication of this study is that providing facilities to accommodate children is a major factor in improving retention and outcome for drug-using mothers in treatment. In addition, having the children in the facility provides opportunities to assess and meet their needs, which may, in turn, affect the mother's prognosis (Hughes, Coletti, Neri, et al., 1995).

A recent national study of individuals in drug-use treatment programs between 1991 and 1993 showed that women who had at least twenty-eight days of treatment, with at least fourteen days in short-term inpatient care, had sharp reductions in their use of illicit drugs, HIV risk behavior, and illegal activities. For instance, 84 percent of the women who were admitted to long-term residential treatment programs admitted using, at intake, illegal drugs every day or at least once a week. Twelve months after treatment, only 28 percent continued to abuse drugs. Women in short-term inpatient treatment also showed significant reductions in illegal drug use one year after their treatment, with 86 percent admitting use at intake and 32 percent reporting use after one year (Hein and Scheier, 1996).

THE FUTURE OF SUBSTANCE ABUSE IN THE UNITED STATES

Because of the historic focus on alcoholism and its prevention and treatment, a social taboo has arisen which has spawned alcohol-free nightclubs and parties known as raves. Although alcohol is not served at these functions, much more potent and dangerous drugs, such as Ecstasy, are used by the patrons. Not only is it difficult to detect the presence of these drugs, it is also difficult to understand the impact on a person's body and brain. This trend will need to be addressed by municipal governments, and parents are going to need education so that they can learn the identifying symptoms associated with these types of drugs.

Proposed Solutions and Strategies

The prohibition model has been the mainstay of the U.S. drug policy since the early 1900s. The basic policy has changed little and continues to result in higher drug use and addiction rates. The major harm that illegal drugs have caused in the United States is the side effects of illegal drug use and acquisition. The most harmful consequence is serving long prison terms for use or selling small amounts of any soft or hard drugs. In the year 2000, almost a million people were in U.S. prisons for some illegal drug offense. Although there is a great deal of support for U.S. policy shifting to a harm-reduction or public-health model, there is no organized support within the U.S. government for moving in this direction.

Because of growing support for medical marijuana (and marijuana buyers' clubs for patients needing it) and the public view that marijuana can be helpful to those suffering from a number of chronic disorders, the antimarijuana forces are slowly losing ground in the United States. Additionally, there is a pressing need to take a different approach to hard-drug users. The state-supported methadone programs were expanded in the later 1990s, and some private groups were running needle-exchange programs, which actually were illegal but were ignored by local authorities. Overall, however, the United States has not turned the corner in stopping or slowing the illegal drug problem in the United States. And, as long as the emphasis is on the prohibition model for controlling drugs, there is little likelihood that the substance-abuse problem in the United States will improve.

CONCLUSION

When U.S. politicians wage war on drugs, it typically means that the fight will be in another country and that the soldiers in the war will be the politicians and civilians in another country, not the United States. Typically, these other countries have been poor and developing countries. The U.S. drug war has left many foreign politicians (but not U.S. politicians), governments, and national economies in shambles and in the hands of criminals—all in our effort to prevent U.S. citizens from using illegal drugs.

At this point in the year 2001, substance-abuse treatment is still in the most primitive stage of development. We can diagnose but, as of yet, we cannot cure addiction. We do know a few interventions that typically work.

We know the longer the addict is off the addictive drug, the more the body recovers from the effects of the drug on the body's equilibrium. Even then, after years of sobriety, an addict can start using his preferred drug again, and in a short time the addict is using daily as much of the drug as he or she was using before.

This phenomenon called addiction and the U.S. response to it during the twentieth century, can be viewed as a Greek comedy. The harder the United States tries to stop the trafficking in illegal drugs, the worse the drug problem becomes in the United States and around the world, and the more widespread the international illegal drug markets become. The Greek tragedy is the all-or-nothing mentality of U.S. politicians and leaders who will settle for nothing less than abstinence. In the process, the U.S. global drug war, which has lasted almost one hundred years, has resulted in struggling Third World countries and many of their people being destroyed. And in the United States, in the name of illegal drug control, civil rights continue to abridged and reduced. In these ways and many others, the U.S. drug wars touch almost everyone.

REFERENCES

Brooner, R.K.; King, V.L.; Kidorf, M.; et al. (1997). Psychiatric and substance use comorbidity among treatment-seeking opioid abusers. *Archives of General Psychiatry 54* (1), 71–80.

Cherrington, E.H. (1920). *The evolution of prohibition in the United States of America*. Westerville, Ohio: American Issue Press.

Colder, C.R.; Lochman, J.E.; and Wells, K.C. (1997). The moderating effects of children's fear and activity level on relations between parenting practices and childhood symptomatology. *Journal of Abnormal and Child Psychology 25*, 251–263.

Dembo, R.; Dertke, M.; LaVoie, L.; Borders, S.; Washburn, M.; and Schmeidler, J. (1987). Physical abuse, sexual victimization, and illicit drug use: A structural analysis among high risk adolescents. *Journal of Adolescence 10*, 13–33.

Dishion, T.J.; Kavanagh, K.; and Kiesner, J. (1998). Prevention of early substance use among high-risk youth: A multiple gating approach to parent interventions. In *National Conference on Drug Abuse Prevention Research: Presentations, Papers, and Recommendations* (pp. 87–100). Washington, D.C.: U.S. Government Printing Office.

Dodge, K.A.; Lochman, J.E.; Harnish, J.D.; et al. (1997). Reactive and proactive aggression in school children and psychiatrically impaired chronically assaultive youth. *Journal of Abnormal Psychology 106* (1), 37–51.

Duncan, S.C.; Duncan, T.E.; Biglan, A.; and Ary, D.V. (1998). Contributions of social context to the development of adolescent substance use: A multivariate latent growth modeling approach. *Drug and Alcohol Dependence 50*, 57–71.

Encarta Desk Encyclopedia. (1998). Microsoft Corporation on CD-ROM.

Fullilove, M.T.; Fullilove, R.E.; Smith, M.; Winkler, K.; Michael, C.; Panzer, P.G.;

and Wallace, R. (1993). Violence, trauma, post-traumatic stress disorder among women drug users. *Journal of Traumatic Stress* 6 (4), 533–543.

Furnas, J.C. (1965). *The life and times of the late demon rum.* New York: Putnam.

Gondolf, E.W. (1995). Alcohol abuse, wife assault, and power needs. *Social Service Review* 69 (2), 274–284.

Hecht, M.; Trost, M.; Bator, R.; and MacKinnon, D. (1997). Ethnicity and gender similarities and differences in drug resistance. *Journal of Applied Communication Research* 25, 1–23.

Hein, D., and Scheier, J. (1996). Trauma and short-term outcome for women in detoxification. *Journal of Substance Abuse Treatment* 13, 227–231.

Hershow, R.C.; Riester, K.A.; Lew, J.; et al. (1997). Increased vertical transmission of human immunodeficiency virus from hepatitis C virus-coinfected mothers. Women and Infants Transmission Study. *Journal of Infectious Diseases* 176, 414–420.

Hughes, P.H.; Coletti, S.D.; Neri, R.L.; et al. (1995). Retaining cocaine-abusing women in a therapeutic community: The effect of a child live-in program. *American Journal of Public Health* 85 (8), 1149–1152.

Internal Revenue Service. (1921, 1966, 1970). Alcohol and tobacco summary statistics. Washington, D.C.: Government Printing Office.

Jackson, C. (1997). Initiation and experimental stages of tobacco and alcohol during late childhood: Relation to peer, parent, and personal risk factors. *Addictive Behaviors* 22, 1–14.

Lee, H. (1963). *How dry we were: Prohibition revisited.* Englewood Cliffs, NJ: Prentice Hall.

McCurdy, K., and Daro, D. (1994). *Current trends in child abuse reporting and fatalities: The results of the 1993 annual fifty state survey.* Chicago: National Committee to Prevent Child Abuse.

Miller, B.A.; Downs, W.R.; and Gondoli, D.M. (1989). Spousal violence among alcoholic women as compared to a random household sample of women. *Journal of Studies on Alcoholism* 50 (6), 533–540.

Riley, Diane. (1998). *Drug and drug policy in Canada: A brief review & commentary.* Ottawa: Canadian Foundation for Drug Policy.

Roy, M. (1988). *Children in the crossfire: Violence in the home: How does it affect our children?* Deerfield Beach, FL: Health Communications.

SAMHSA [Substance Abuse and Mental Health Services Administration] (1998). *Preliminary results from the 1997 national household survey on drug abuse.* DHHS Pub. No. (SMA) 98–3200. Rockville, MD: Author. Also available electronically at www.samhsa.gov or at www.health.org, pp. 9–14.

Scheier, L.M.; Botvin, G.J.; and Baker, E. (1997). Risk and protective factors as predictors of adolescent alcohol involvement and transition in alcohol use: A prospective analysis. *Journal of Alcohol Studies* 58 (6); 652–667.

Sinclair, A. (1962). *The era of excess.* Boston: Little, Brown.

Sloboda, Zila, and David, Susan. (2000). *Preventing drug use among children and adolescents: A research guide.* Bethesda, Maryland: The National Institute of Drug Abuse.

Stacy, A.W.; Galaif, E.; Sussman, S.; and Dent, C.W. (1996). Self-generated drug outcomes in continuation high school students. *Psychology of Addictive Behaviors* 10, 18–27.

Stark, E., and Flitcraft, A. (1988). Violence among intimates: An epidemiological review. In V.D. Van Hasselt, R.L. Morrison, A.S. Bellack, and M. Herson (Eds.), *Handbook of Family Violence*. (pp. 159–199). New York: Plenum.

Timberlake, J.H. (1963). *Prohibition and the progressive movement*. Cambridge: Harvard University Press.

U.S. Department of Health and Human Services. (1997). *Substance abuse treatment and domestic violence, treatment improvement protocol (TIP)*, Series 25. DHHS Publication no. (SMA) 97–3163. Washington, D.C.: Government Printing Office.

POSTSCRIPT

One way to understand people with drug or alcohol addiction is to imagine them as being disabled and in need of continued care. Treatment for a disability should be designed to work closely with and accept chronic relapses. Addiction is a horrible disorder, and it can be very disabling; however, it is preventable, and it does not have to be so destructive. Which is more harmful, drug use and addiction or spending years in prison as an addict? When treating an addict, therapists are not concerned about a drug being legal or illegal. The only difference is that using an illegal drug, in addition to its being addictive, can result in the addict's becoming a criminal justice statistic.

Stressful surroundings can increase hopelessness, anxiety, and depression. Poverty is a major cause of overall stress for an individual and a family. People seek relief from the distress. If drugs are readily available and if they are perceived to reduce the stress, many people will use them despite the risk. Often the media tap into the stresses of life and depict drugs as a carefree way to seek relief. For instance, alcohol is depicted as an enjoyable way to meet attractive people of the opposite sex, and beauty is portrayed as being anorexic, similar to the way people look when they use large amounts of heroin or crack cocaine. Young girls and boys are most susceptible to persuasion by the media.

Another contributing condition that places young people at risk for drug use is the ban on drugs, which creates an attractive mystique. Criminalizing drugs has a number of adverse effects on young people. Information becomes suppressed when people begin to use and traffic drugs illegally.

Therefore, over time, the general public and policy makers fail to make informed decisions on the future course of society. As more of the older generations of addicts are placed in jail, younger generations do not receive the full picture of the problem, so it becomes easier to believe the glamorization from the media and peers. When a public health approach is used to deal with addiction, it will do less harm and more good than a criminal justice model. This approach must include prevention and education programs to reduce the number of future addicts.

INDEX

ABOUT THE EDITORS
AND CONTRIBUTORS

ANDREW CHERRY is a Professor of Social Work at Barry University, Miami, Florida.

MARY E. DILLON is a doctorate candidate at Nova University, School of Education, Ft. Lauderdale, Florida, and the Executive Director of Biscayne Institute, Miami, Florida.

DOUGLAS RUGH is a doctoral candidate at Florida International University, School of Social Work, Miami, Florida.

LOUIS B. ANTOINE is an Assistant Professor of Clinical Psychiatry at the University of Miami, School of Medicine, Miami, Florida.

IRENE MOREDA is a Professor of Social Work at Barry University, Miami, Florida.

KATHRYN C. SHAFER is an Assistant Professor of Social Work at the University of South Florida, Tampa, Florida.